To Ashley

Thank you for caring

Chuck Rome

2022

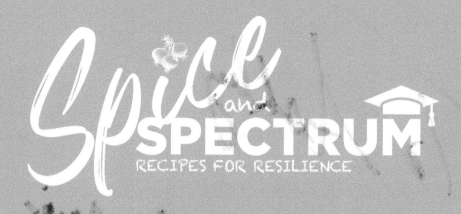

Spice and SPECTRUM
RECIPES FOR RESILIENCE

PROSPERITY PUBLICATIONS, LLC
San Antonio, TX
www.prosperitypublications.com

iCAN DREAM CENTER https://icandreamcenter.com

ISBN: 2370001645721

Cover Design: Hilary Rhodes Designs
Layout: Pixel Munki | JR Arthur
Printed by: Trevett's Printing, Irmo, SC

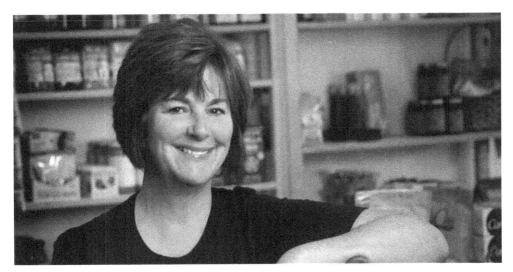

FOREWORD

As the owner of Dunning's Market, I spend a lot of time thinking about food.

What some of you may not know is I have a son with autism, so I also spend a lot of time thinking about how we as a community can better serve kids on the spectrum.

That's why I am so happy to have this book at the intersection of good food and great kids who are so often overlooked. All the recipes you'll find in Spice & Spectrum were tested in the kitchen by neurodiverse young adults.

This book was developed by Chef Jerome Brown, known for his impressive culinary skills and his big heart - he gives his time and energy to raise money for programming at the iCan Dream Center, a not-for-profit therapeutic school serving students with various learning deficits in the south suburbs of Chicago.

This cookbook is so special - all the recipes are delicious and easy to follow. They are for everyone but adapted with an eye toward straight forward ease.

So, dig in and get cooking! Try out the recipes and tell us how you liked them and what you did to give them your own special signature! We hope they move you as much as they did us. And please remind everyone you know to pick up a copy so that we can help make the future better and brighter for the students at the iCan Dream Center and beyond!

Maureen Mader
Owner and Operator of Dunning's Market

BASKING IN GRATITUDE

This project has made my heart overflow with gratitude and has come to fruition in a manner that I could not have imagined. Firstly, I thank God for entrusting me with the vision for His beloved. The Lord constantly provides resources and divine connections to make this vision a reality. The way the pieces of this cookbook came together has left me in awe. I began following a few celebrity chefs to find the right one for this cookbook project that was on my heart, and I finally found Chef Rome on Instagram. It had been months since I had interacted with anyone or even looked at their social media presence. Chef Jerome's Instagram account was hacked in August 2020. This provided me with the opportunity to alert him to this project. A couple weeks later, we met in Mexico (where he was working and I was on vacation), and he enthusiastically agreed to partner with me. I have never seen his enthusiasm wane since that day. I am forever grateful for all the time and effort he has put into this project. Chef Rome has become a trusted friend, confidant, and a great supporter of iCan Dream Center! We love you; you are family now.

Zipporah, Your love leaves no heart untouched. You are so much more than a Culinary Coordinator, Chaplain, CPR Trainer, or Behavior Specialist—you are a culture curator. You are the embodiment of my greatest hope for our organization's culture. Thank you for your kindness toward our students, the team, and me. This project would not have been possible without you.

My dear **Katie**, I am so glad that God allowed our paths to cross and that you have joined the iCan Dream family. This project has been elevated by your passion in ways I could never have imagined. With a remarkable sense of decorum, you bring out the best in everyone. Throughout the process, you have been our chief encourager, creative director, and role model for self-care. Thanks to you, this project took shape, and I am ever grateful for your contributions.

Nikki, I am fortunate to call you my friend, my sister, and the person who always manages to make me laugh effortlessly. It was your humor that kept me afloat during some very difficult moments that could have threatened the success of this project. I am grateful for your contribution to this book; I have always enjoyed reading your work. Furthermore, I am grateful that you love me enough to provide me with honest feedback. The gift of your authenticity is priceless to me.

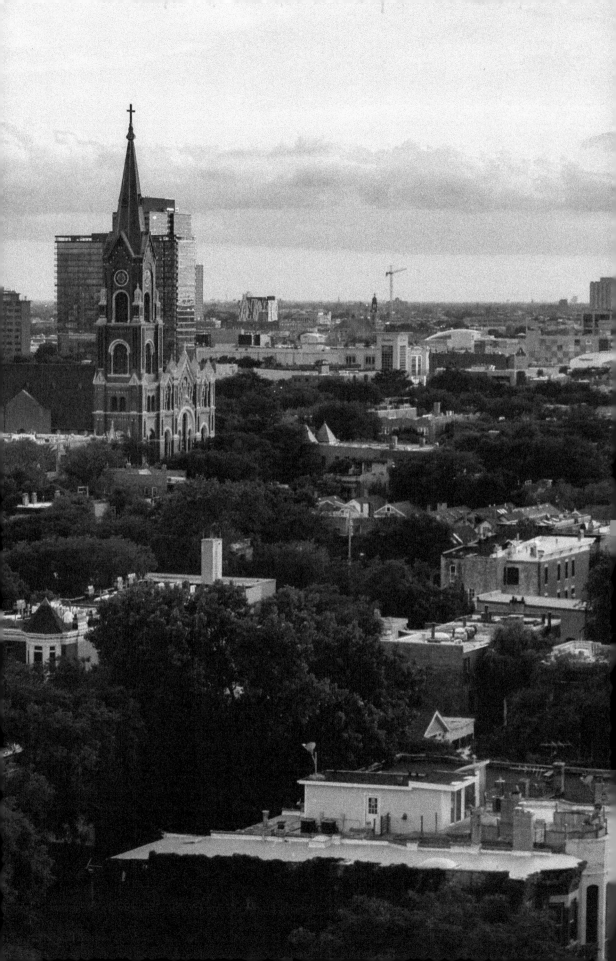

Thank you for your generosity, **JR**. Thank you for catching the vision and providing us with so much more than we expected. The impact of **Pixel Munki** will be felt forever at the iCan Dream Center.

Thank you to **Hilary Rhodes Design** and **Hilary Rhodes**! Thank you for bearing with us during our dreaming sessions and for helping us create pure beauty.

We value the trust you place in us, parents, and district leaders. These precious students, who are the focus of this cookbook, have been entrusted to us by you. It is our pleasure to work with you.

We would like to thank the **iCan Dream Center family** for fostering creativity in our students, creating a comfortable setting for them to tell their stories, and for capturing those special moments. It is thanks to you all that our learners can make sense of their pain and clarify their dreams. Thank you for showing up every day to support young people in their pursuit of purpose.

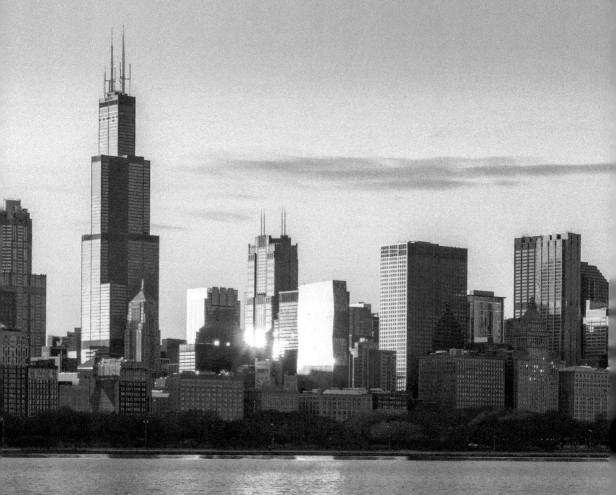

66 Previously stated that I was done writing cookbooks. It's a tedious task to say the least, and I was certain that I was all but done with the notion. However, I'm grateful to have this opportunity to have cooked up something special in Chicago that gives so much to those who are open to receive it. 99

A NOTE FROM ROME

It's amazing to me how life's special moments come together. The moment Dr. Ford asked me to be a part of this amazing project, I knew I needed to first educate myself. I've learned so much in this short period of time. Having a sister with a developmental disability, I realized that there's more that I still need to know as I had never known or been around anyone with autism prior to now.

The opportunity to visit the iCan Dream Center and prepare recipes from this book provided a way for me to interact with the students and learn from them. I have to say they poured into me. I will never forget the day one of the students said to me that he had never tasted steak before. As we prepared the stove top steak recipe, I knew I would send one home with him so that he could enjoy a juicy steak that he had assisted in the preparation of. It gave me a sense of happiness that I could do something to brighten up his day, just as those students have brightened up my life. I'm grateful for Dr. Ford and the iCan Dream Center staff, as well as the students, for all their support in making this cookbook come to life.

I had previously stated that I was done writing cookbooks. It's a tedious task to say the least, and I was certain that I was all but done with the notion. However, I'm grateful to have this opportunity to have cooked up something special in Chicago that gives so much to those who are open to receive it.

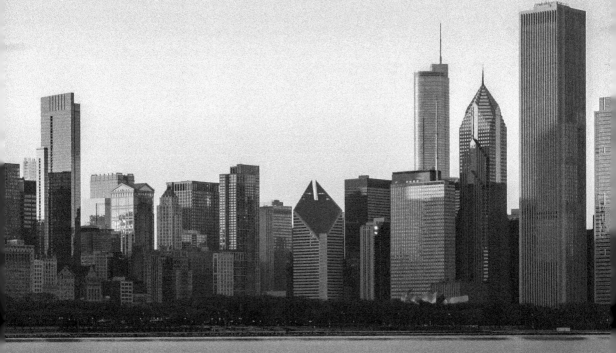

TABLE OF CONTENTS

AMPLIFY | 69

MOBILIZE | 113

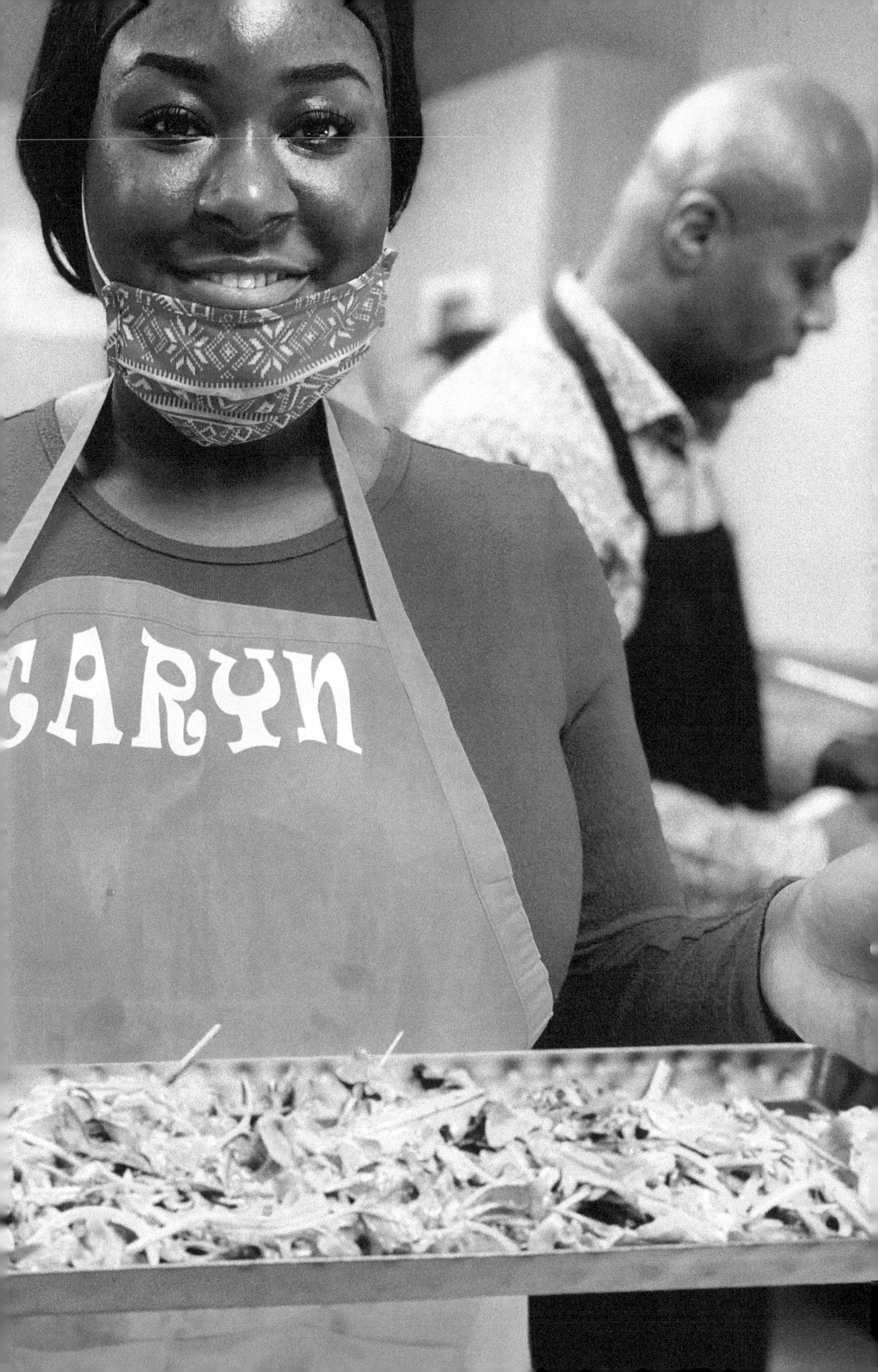
ARYN

DREAM

As an administrator of special education programs in a public school, I developed several programs to meet the needs of students with disabilities. Whenever I recognize an opportunity to serve students better, I never ignore it. It was during my five-year tenure as the director of special education in the school district where I was hired that I developed or revamped five programs.

In my doctoral studies, I chose to study the most effective programmatic features to facilitate success for students with disabilities. In my school district (at the time), I discovered a critical gap in services for students who were not on track to graduate. These students were at risk of being involved in the criminal justice system. Even though this is not the responsibility of the school district per se, this group of students touched my heart. These were the students whose parents I had to look at across the table at expulsion hearings so many times. Moreover, these were the students who may have been encouraged to enroll in a GED program, which is akin to being asked to drop out of high school because the completion rate is so low that it is laughable. Despite obtaining a diploma, these students would end up sitting on the couch playing video games, browsing social media, or engaging in more dangerous activities due to the conditioning they acquired from previous traumatic experiences. It is true that this is a group of students that the district would do well to wash their hands of, but they kept me awake many nights. Therefore, I set about developing a program that would address their needs.

By developing a staffing plan, the district was able to save money. Among my goals was to obtain space donated to the college because I believed it was important to give students a sense of dignity; they needed a space that was not intended for secondary students since that environment had not been successful for them. In addition, I developed a partnership with the community college to provide the students with a diploma, transitional skills, and vocational training. I was delighted to share my developments with the superintendent. When he halted my plans to develop an appropriate program because the district was in the middle of a teacher contract negotiation, I was stunned. The fact that this program would benefit minority students disproportionately felt to some like an obstacle to overcome, rather than an opportunity. Observing the reasons given to me, none of which seemed persuasive, my heart broke for those students who felt like an afterthought of this bureaucratic process.

A short time later, I was attending a church service and one thing that was said by the guest speaker during the message still resonates in my soul: "If you see the need, that is the call." And in that moment, I began to **DREAM** for these marginalized students. To improve my original program, I began to think outside of the confines of the public school system. This program was intended to manifest in an entirely different context. In the following months, with my stomach in my throat, I submitted a letter of resignation.

With its founding in March 2013, iCan Dream Center has served as a midwife to hundreds of students whose dreams were brought to life by individuals who saw and recognized their potential. The focus of this cookbook is on the potential of students. This program is an example of how iCan Dream Center reduces the barriers that are far too often present for students who are systemically forgotten.

Discover how we provide our youth with new opportunities so that they can thrive within the community by joining us on our journey. There is much work to be done to foster a barrier-free society. However, we are committed to making a positive contribution. Therefore, at iCan Dream Center, and on these pages, we have created a platform where youth can meaningfully participate and contribute. Come cook with us! You will find recipes on these pages that will nourish your body, as well as stories of our youth that will nourish your soul.

Dr. Evisha Ford

Dr. Evisha Ford
Founder & Executive Director of iCan Dream Center, NFP

We fuel **dreams** by **empowering youth** and their **families** with the **skills** to **thrive.**

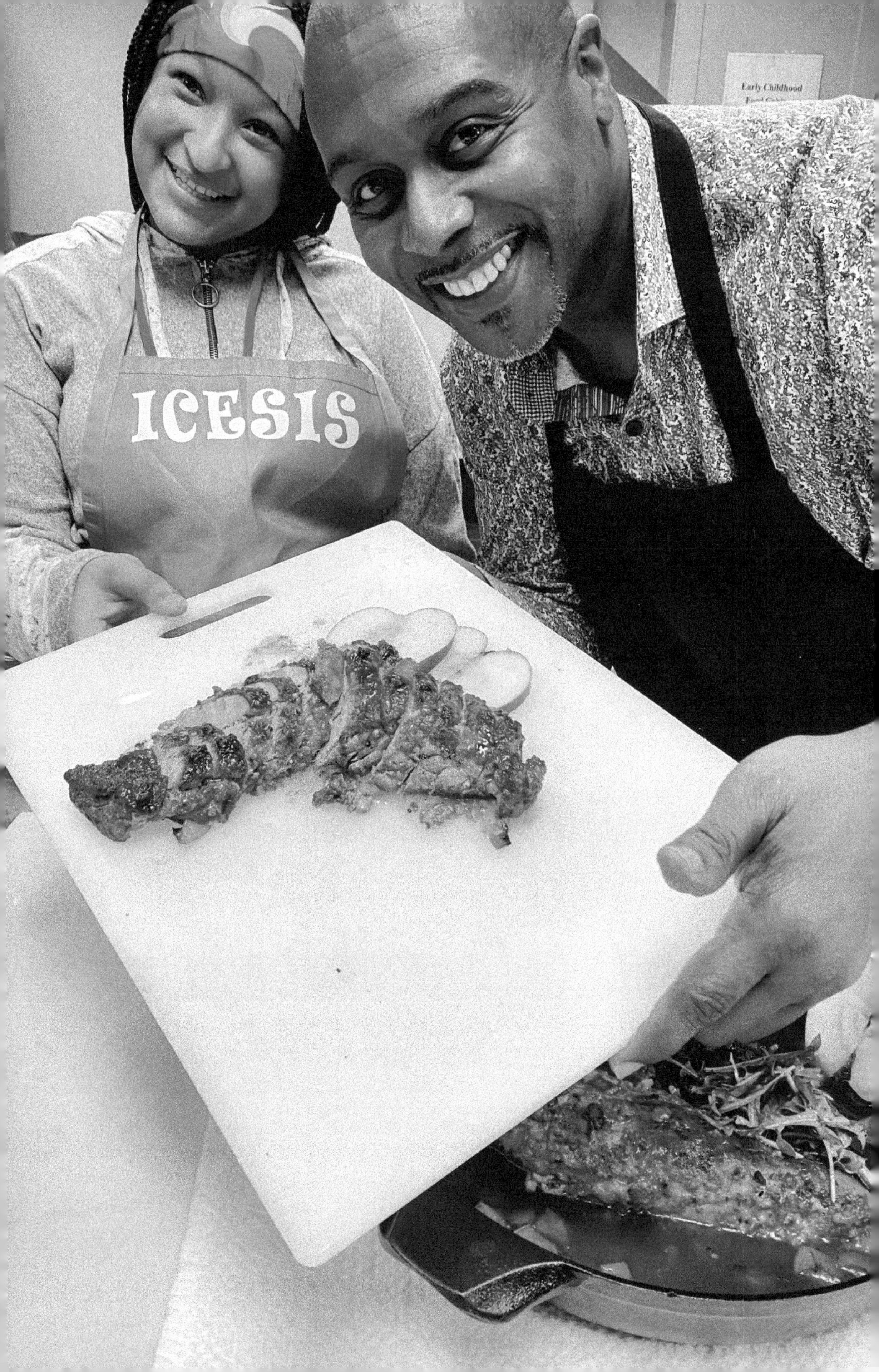
Early Childhood
ICESIS

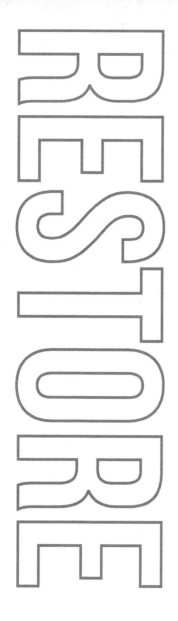

RESTORE

To enhance one's daily life, promote wellness, and longevity, healthy eating must become a lifestyle.

Israeli Couscous & Kale Salad

Lemon Basil Vinaigrette

Veggie Mostaccioli

Rainbow Potatoes

Grilled Parmesan Roasted Asparagus with Balsamic Glaze

Penne Pasta & Brussel Sprouts

Bok Choy Saute

Oven Roasted Lemon Pepper Trout & Lemon Garlic Sauce

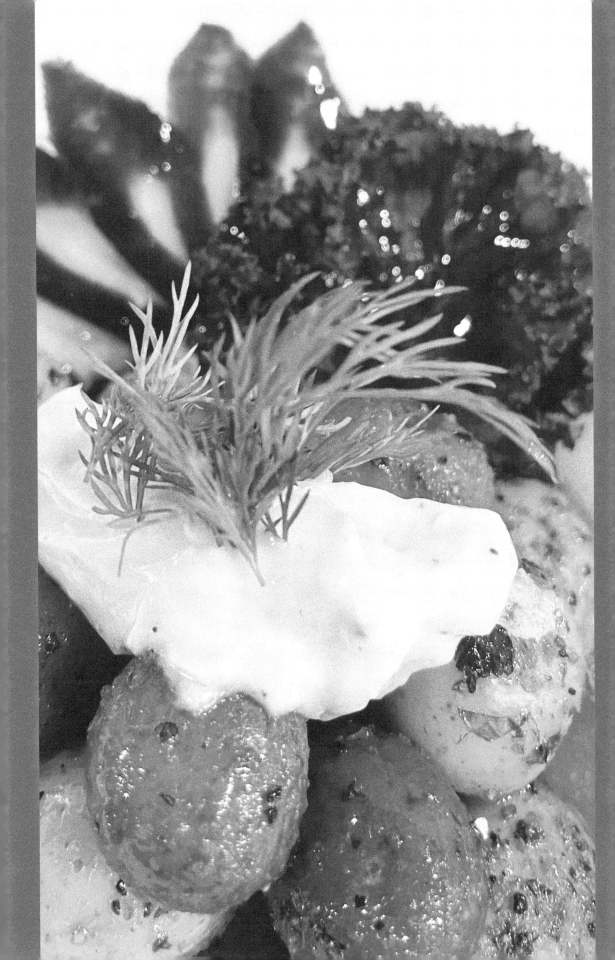

RESTORE

Healthful eating must become a lifestyle to improve one's health, well-being, and longevity. Exercise and diet are two of the most important aspects of health and wellness. Even the healthiest people can fall victim to cravings, or lapses in judgment when it comes to snacking and overeating. There is no need to worry, we are all human. In our case, the human body has remarkable restorative and detoxification abilities which can either be hindered or greatly enhanced by the food we choose to consume to assist in protecting our health when certain foods have compromised our health. We heal ourselves with our food, and our food is our medicine.

The importance of taking notice, and even making accommodations when sharing the table with children, especially those with developmental or intellectual disabilities, cannot be overstated. According to research, people with disabilities tend to suffer from more gut disorders, sensitivities, and food intolerances. Often, these issues are related to sensory obstacles, where texture competes with taste. It is important to understand that diet should not be confused with the latest trends on how to lose weight, which assumes that size and weight are the only indicators of what it means to be healthy. However, appearances are not always indicative of health. In our society, it may pay to appear good, however, our values are terribly misplaced; nutrition is far more valuable, and sometimes very costly. We are thus left with a dilemma that can sometimes deter us from eating, feeling, and ultimately leading a healthy life.

The ability to afford a healthier lifestyle should not be a luxury. It is important to note that such a diet is accessible to all and does not always require the most expensive organic foods. It is quite possible for most of us to fuel the body toward health using creativity, a little education, and a little ingenuity. These days, a growing number of discount stores offer healthier alternatives, including fruits, vegetables, whole grains, lean proteins, nuts, and seeds. Since organics have become a mainstream product, they are easier to find and less expensive than in the past. Making simple changes, such as replacing canned vegetables with frozen ones, consuming fewer processed foods, and eating more fresh foods, can have a significant impact on your eating habits, and therefore, your life.

Those of us who may suffer from mental or physical imbalance can greatly benefit from becoming more mindful of what we put into the **RESTORE** body.

A healthy diet may not seem as appetizing as eating a hamburger and fries, however, depending on the ingredients of the burger, eating one can be a healthy option. For example, whole grain buns restore the body, while white bread provides little benefit. As well as the difference between grass-fed and factory farmed meats and cheese compared to no cheese. There can be an important difference between a healthy and a nutritionally dense hamburger. It is easy to prepare healthy French fries by slicing a potato and roasting it or sautéing it in olive oil and they will probably taste better than the frozen ones that cost twice as much.

There is no doubt that food has the power to reverse sickness, combat aging, and improve cognition and mental health. Researchers have found that certain types of food can promote a healthier microbiome in the gut, and when the digestive system is in the healthiest of states, the mind will also be; and the body will follow. Foods that are less natural are more toxic to the body. It is an inherent function of the human body to discern what is compatible and what is not, and allergies are a prime example of our bodies rejecting toxins, yet we continue to consume unhealthy foods.

In the modern world, our taste buds have been hijacked and it has become more difficult to distinguish between what tastes good and what is healthy. Having a diet rich in nutrients is an important factor in maintaining good health. Unfortunately, nutrition is sold as a commodity in our society, and it is up to us to determine what is healthy. Knowing better makes it easier for us to make wise choices. Thus, here are some suggestions to add to your grocery list, or to replace items that replenish the body. We should consider the oils we consume and begin to experiment with healthier fats, such as coconut oil, avocados, ghee, and olive oil. It is important to limit the use of highly processed oils such as corn, soybean, and canola oils. Sugar, especially artificial sugars, and high fructose corn syrup should absolutely be avoided. If sweet is necessary, consider raw honey, agave nectar, dates, monk fruit, and cacao for chocolate lovers. Many would argue that it is best to avoid milk altogether; however, if necessary, some alternatives include almond, cashew, hemp, and many others. As an alternative, oat milk is available, although it is not recommended for those who are gluten sensitive. It is recommended that beans, nuts, and seeds be soaked prior to consumption. Soy should not be consumed. Mushrooms are an excellent and healthy alternative to meat. Mushrooms and honey products are often used medicinally (unless you are allergic). Garlic, ginger, lemon, oregano, rosemary, parsley, and cilantro are some of the other ingredients. In addition to food rich in color, foods rich in antioxidants, which are naturally occurring, are the very best. The best way to get the most out of these foods could be to blend them all together into a smoothie instead of drinking artificially flavored juice or soda. Even water that has been sprinkled with a small amount of pink or Celtic salt is packed with minerals and is far superior to table salt that has been bleached. Yuck!

Consuming whole foods greatly improves one's health by supporting the immune system, promoting physical and mental wellbeing, as well as improving cognitive function. Holistically, it is more important to eat a balanced diet rather than strictly organic. Another term to become familiar with is non-GMO, and reading labels is another skill that should be learned.

> **" In most cultures, eating is a meaningful bonding experience, but for families with neurodiverse family members who struggle at mealtime, eating can be more of a challenge. "**

It is important to become informed about what we consume, model healthy behaviors, and to share this knowledge with family and friends to promote generational health and quality of life. In most cultures, eating is a meaningful bonding experience, but for families with neurodiverse family members who struggle at mealtime, eating can be more of a challenge. To introduce new foods to a child's palate both for variety's sake, as well as to provide a balanced diet, creativity and imagination will be required. Remember that what might be delicious to one person may not be to another. For example, avocado mashed potatoes are delicious! Here is a list of the fruits and vegetables that one should purchase organically. If organic foods are not available to you, it is still better to consume a diet rich in fruits and vegetables over processed packaged food and junk food. After all, you are what you eat. Bon Appetit!

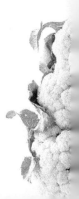

THE DIRTY DOZEN

1. Strawberries
2. Spinach
3. Kale/Collard/Mustard Greens
4. Nectarines
5. Apples
6. Grapes
7. Cherries
8. Peaches
9. Pears
10. Bell & Hot Peppers
11. Celery
12. Tomatoes

CLEAN 15

1. Avocados
2. Sweet Corn
3. Pineapples
4. Onions
5. Papayas
6. Frozen Sweet Peas
7. Eggplant
8. Asparagus
9. Broccoli
10. Cabbage
11. Kiwifruit
12. Cauliflower
13. Mushrooms
14. Honeydew
15. Cantaloupe

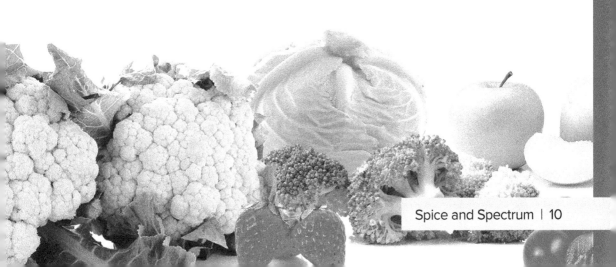

ISRAELI COUSCOUS & KALE SALAD

Serves: 8

INGREDIENTS

COUSCOUS
2 Tablespoon of olive oil

2 Cups of Israeli couscous

4 Cups of water

VEGETABLE SAUTÉ
4 Tablespoons of Olive oil

1 White onion *(chopped)*

4 Cloves of garlic *(chopped)*

1 Red bell pepper *(chopped)*

2 Cups of kale leaves
(rough chopped)

DRESSING
1 Cup of white wine vinegar

2 Tablespoons of sugar

Pinch of salt

Dash of black pepper

2 Tablespoons of olive oil

DIRECTIONS

Place a medium pot onto the stove on medium high. Add the oil and allow it to heat up. Add the couscous to the pan and sauté for about 2 minutes. Add the water and bring to a boil. Cook for about 10 minutes or until done. Drain the couscous. Run under cold-water to help the couscous to cool off. Place into the refrigerator to chill until further use.

Place a large skillet onto the stove on medium high. Add the oil, garlic, bell pepper and kale. Cook for about 4 minutes. Remove the mix from the stove and place into a bowl. Set aside for later use.

To create the dressing, combine all the ingredients in a blender. Blend on high for about 5 seconds.

Combine all the couscous, vegetables, and dressing together. Chill until ready to serve.

Toss well and serve. Enjoy!

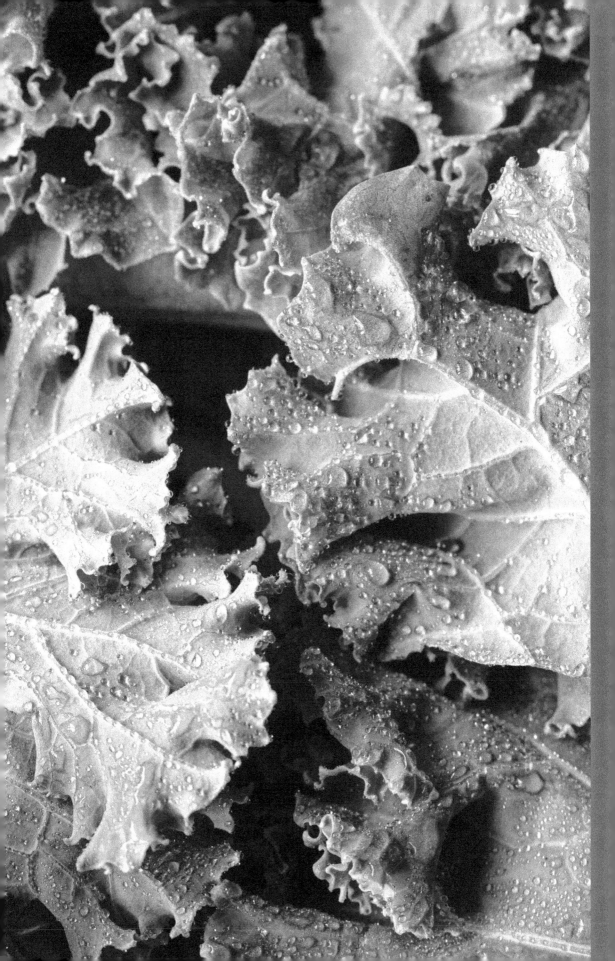

LEMON BASIL VINAIGRETTE

Serves: 4

INGREDIENTS

1 Shallot *(chopped)*

1 Teaspoon of minced garlic

Juice of 1 lemon

Zest of 1 lemon

Pinch of crushed red pepper flakes

Pinch of salt

2 Tablespoons of sugar

½ Tablespoon of chopped basil

½ Cup of white wine vinegar

¼ Cup of olive oil

DIRECTIONS

Combine all the ingredients in a blender. Pulse for about 5 seconds. Store in a plastic container with a tight-fitting lid. Use when ready.

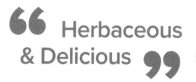

" Herbaceous & Delicious "

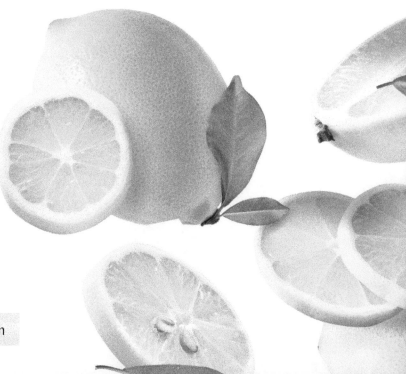

OVEN ROASTED LEMON PEPPER TROUT & LEMON GARLIC SAUCE

Serves: 4

INGREDIENTS

4 Fresh trout
(dressed and butterflied)

1 Stick of melted butter

1 Tablespoon of olive oil

Juice of one lemon

Zest of one lemon

¼ Cup of veggie broth

1 Tablespoon of Dijon mustard

1 Teaspoon of lemon
pepper seasoning

1 Tablespoon of chopped
parsley *(fresh)*

LEMON GARLIC SAUCE

1 Tablespoon of sliced
butter *(salted)*

4 Garlic cloves

Juice of one freshly
squeezed lemon

Pinch of smoked paprika

2 Tablespoon of heavy cream

DIRECTIONS

Preheat your oven to 425. Place a large cast iron skillet onto the stove on medium high. In a small mixing bowl, combine the melted butter, oil, lemon juice, zest, veggie broth, and mustard. Mix well. Using a spatula, spread the mixture over flesh side of the fish. Place the fish into the skillet and add the remaining ingredients to the fish. Place the fish into the oven and finish cooking for about 10 minutes. Remove the fish from the oven and place back onto the stove. Place the fish onto a platter. Garnish with lemon slices and fresh parsley.

LEMON GARLIC SAUCE – After removing the fish from the stove, Place the skillet back on the stove. Add to the skillet the butter, garlic, lemon juice, paprika, and heavy cream. Bring to a simmer. Pour the sauce over the fish. Enjoy!

VEGGIE MOSTACCIOLI

Serves: 10

INGREDIENTS

1 Box of mostaccioli pasta

1 Tablespoon of salt

2 Tablespoons of vegetable oil

½ Eggplant *(diced)*

10 Broccoli crowns

8oz. of mushrooms

1 Zucchini *(small diced)*

1 Onion *(diced)*

1 Tablespoon of minced garlic

1 Tablespoon of marinara sauce

1 Tablespoon of sugar

2 Tablespoons of olive oil

2 Cups of Monterey Jack cheese

DIRECTIONS

Pre-heat the oven on 400. Place a large pot of water on the stove on high. Allow the water to come to a boil. Add the salt and pasta to the water. Cook the pasta according to the directions on the package. Place a strainer in the sink and pour in the pasta. Drain and run under cold water to stop the cooking of the pasta. Add the olive oil and mix well. Set aside until ready for use.

Place a large skillet onto the stove on medium high. Add the vegetable oil to the pan along with the diced and chopped vegetables. Sauté for about 5 minutes. Add the marinara and sugar to the vegetables. Add the pasta to the vegetables and mix well.

Place the pasta and vegetables into a casserole dish. Top with cheese. Cover with foil and bake for 30 minutes. Remove the foil. Add extra cheese or Mozzarella *(optional)*. Continue to bake until the cheese is golden brown.

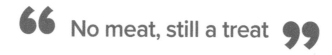

No meat, still a treat

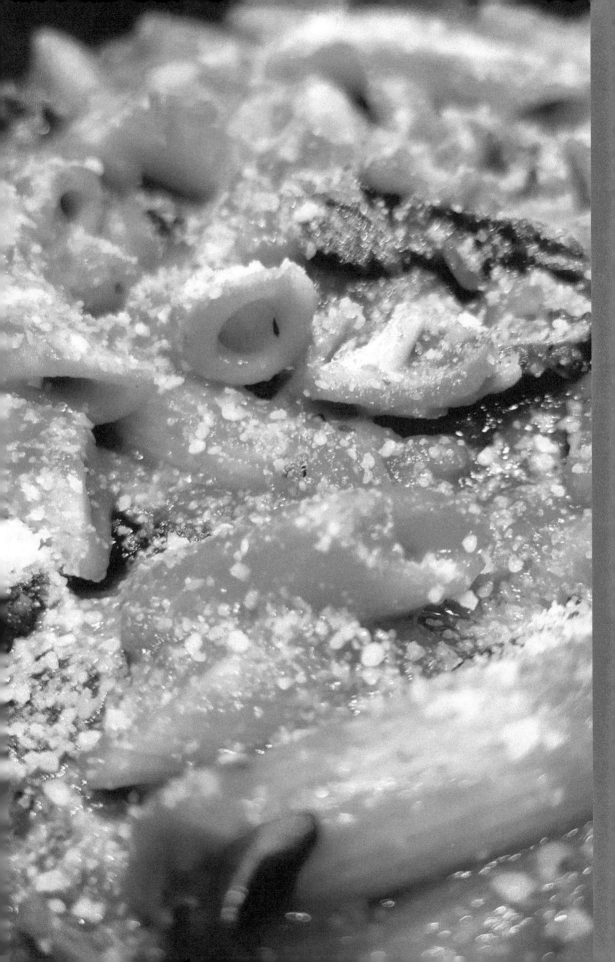

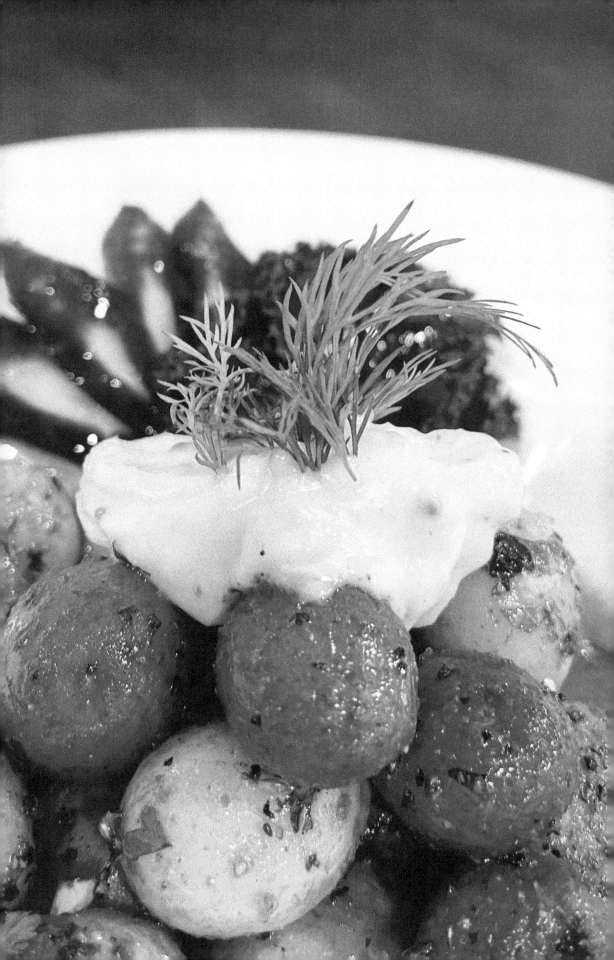

RAINBOW POTATOES

Serves: 4 – 6

INGREDIENTS

1 Pound of baby potatoes *(red, white, and purple)*

½ Quart of vegetable broth

1 Teaspoon of dry thyme

1 Tablespoon of chopped parsley

1 Tablespoon of fresh chopped rosemary

2 Teaspoons of seasoned salt

1 Teaspoon of garlic powder

¼ Cup of olive oil

1 Tablespoon of butter *(unsalted)*

DIRECTIONS

In a medium pot, rinse the potatoes off well until they are free from dirt. Pour the vegetable broth over the potatoes. Allow the potatoes to come to a boil. Reduce the heat to low and allow the potatoes to simmer until fork tender. Check the potatoes after 10 minutes. In the meantime, place a skillet on the stove on medium high. Once the potatoes are done, pour the water off the potatoes. Add the oil and butter to the skillet. Add the potatoes into the skillet and sauté for about 2 minutes. Sprinkle the parmesan over the potatoes and serve.

 Somewhere over the potato

GRILLED PARMESAN ROASTED ASPARAGUS WITH BALSAMIC GLAZE

Serves: 4

INGREDIENTS

1 Pound of thick asparagus
(thin works just as well)

1 Tablespoon of olive oil

2 Tablespoons of melted butter
(unsalted)

1 Tablespoon of granulated garlic

2 Teaspoons of black pepper

½ Cup of parmesan cheese

¼ Cup of balsamic vinegar

2 Teaspoons of lite brown sugar

DIRECTIONS

Place a grated cast iron skillet onto the stove on medium high. Rinse the asparagus under cold water. Drain well. Place the asparagus into the skillet. Add the olive oil and butter. Season with the garlic and pepper. Cook for about 3 minutes. Transfer the asparagus to a platter. Sprinkle with parmesan cheese.

In a small sauce pot, add the vinegar and brown sugar. Allow the sauce to warm and mix well. Drizzle the sauce over the asparagus and enjoy.

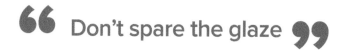

66 Don't spare the glaze **99**

PENNE PASTA & BRUSSELS SPROUTS

Serves: 8

INGREDIENTS

1 Pound of penne pasta

Pinch of salt

1 Tablespoon of vegetable oil

4 Strips of center cut bacon *(chopped) (optional)*

½ Pound of fresh Brussels sprouts (thin sliced

½ Cup of sliced mushrooms

½ Yellow onion *(thin sliced)*

1 Teaspoon of cracked black pepper

½ Cup of grated parmesan cheese

DIRECTIONS

Prepare the pasta according to the directions on the package. Add a pinch of salt to the water once its boiling. Add the pasta into the pot and stir well to prevent from sticking. Once the pasta is done, drain well. Add the vegetable oil to the pasta and toss well. Set aside for later use.

Place a large skillet onto the stove on medium high. Add the bacon to the pan. Cook until the bacon is crispy. Remove the bacon from the pan. Add sprouts, mushrooms, onion and black pepper to the skillet and sauté for about 5 minutes. Add the pasta into the pan and continue to cook until the pasta is back up to temperature. Spoon the pasta onto a platter or plate. Top with parmesan cheese.

BOK CHOY SAUTE'

Serves: 4

INGREDIENTS

2 Strips of chopped bacon
*(use 2 tablespoons of vegetable oil
for those who don't eat pork)*

1 Small chopped onion

2 Tablespoons of unsalted butter

Pinch of crushed red
pepper flakes

8 Baby Bok Choy

1 Tablespoon of
rotisserie seasoning

½ Tablespoon of garlic powder

Juice of ½ lime

DIRECTIONS

Place a large skillet on the stove on medium high. Allow the skillet to heat up for about 5 minutes. Place the chopped bacon and onion into the skillet. Cook the bacon until it's crispy. Remove the bacon from the pan and set aside for garnish. Add the butter and red pepper flakes to the skillet along with the Bok Choy. Sauté for about 4 minutes. Add the remaining ingredients and continue cooking for an additional 3 minutes. Serve as an amazing side or enjoy as a great vegetarian dish.

NOTE: *The bacon can be substituted with vegetable or olive oil.*

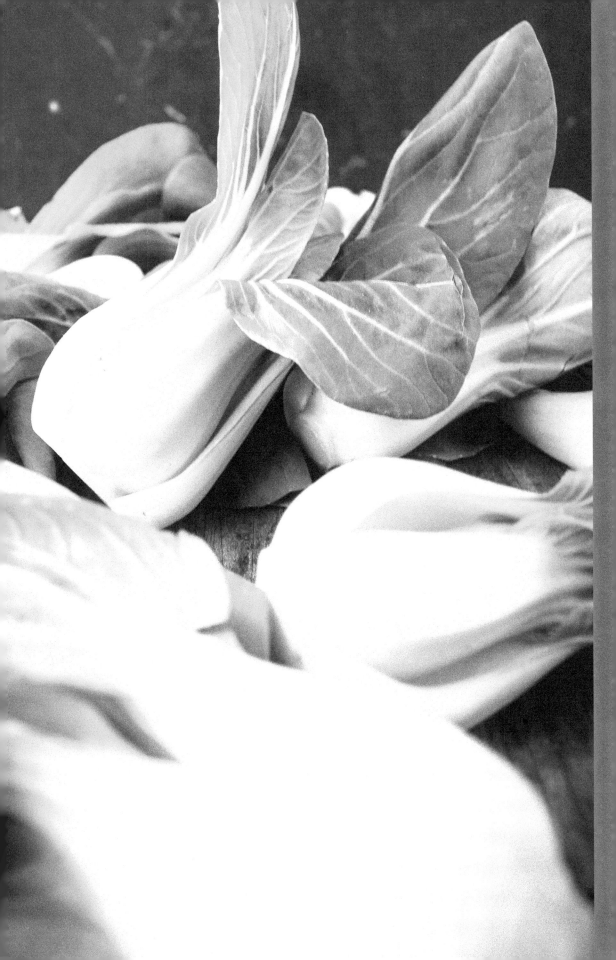

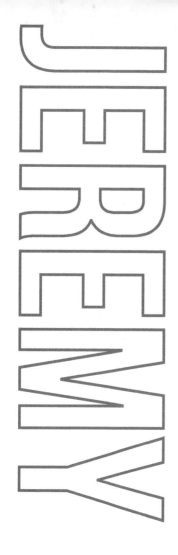

JEREMY

During culinary classes, students practice various academic skills such as basic math as they count, weigh, measure, and keep track of time.

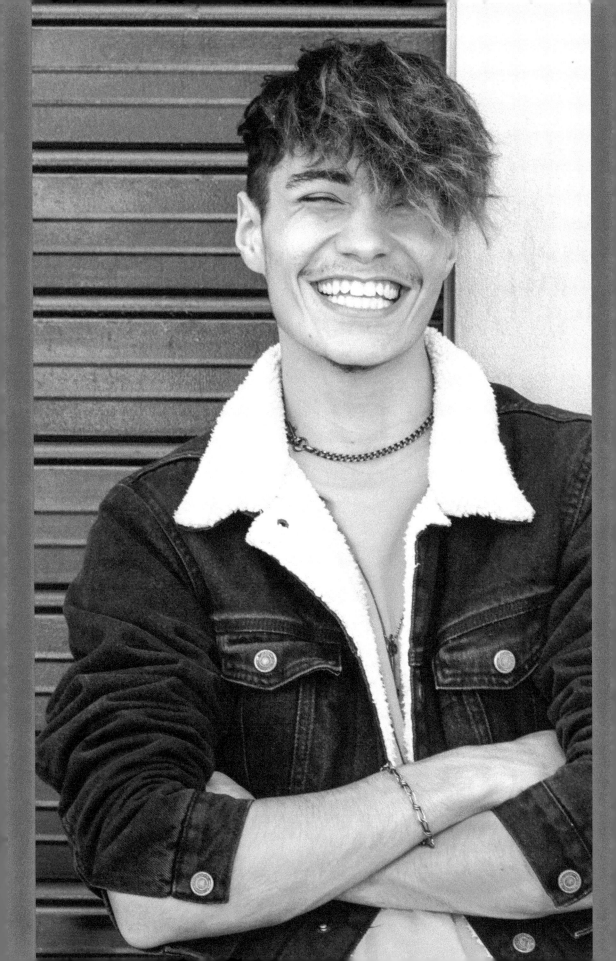

JEREMY

Teenagers and young adults can develop unhealthy eating habits. Cooking classes, on the other hand, get students excited about healthy recipes and the cooking process. Consequently, many teens become interested in eating healthier.

Jeremy was a 17-year-old high school junior who loved French fries and soda when he came to iCan Dream Center. Jeremy is currently 21 years old and a student in our transition program for 18-22-year-olds. He has had many years of culinary training. Chef Jerome came to the center to introduce the students to gourmet cuisine, and Jeremy recalled that over the years, his eating habits had changed from craving salty fried food to the more flavorful and fresh food that Ms. Zipporah taught him. Jeremy has a newfound appreciation for the benefits that better food has on his body, from salmon and rice to spaghetti and salad.

While our culinary students are always served healthy, nutritious food, that doesn't mean they are strangers to Ms. Z's famous peach cobbler or her homemade caramel muffins. Many students need to learn about balance and the lesson has been retained by Jeremy. By making better food choices and trying out new dishes that he would not have attempted at home, Jeremy has been able to lead a healthier lifestyle and to expand his social experiences with food. However, healthy eating is not everything. As students count, weigh, measure, and keep track of time during culinary classes, they practice various academic skills, including basic math. Biology (where food comes from) and chemistry (how high temperatures can alter the composition of food or how the structure of the yolk changes as it is whipped) are taught to the students. Through cooking classes, students also develop social skills by working in teams and communicating with each other. Additionally, students become acquainted with kitchen equipment and cooking technologies.

Cooking classes are not by accident used to increase the self-confidence of youth. Students feel accomplished when they are cooking. When students see the tangible results of their efforts, they feel satisfied. Therefore, some of them can cook at home, assist their parents in the kitchen routine, and even express their opinions. We find that cooking improves the work ethic of people.

Because students with disabilities are entrusted with a variety of tasks in the kitchen related not just to cooking, but also to safety and cleanup, they develop a sense of responsibility. We observe that our students become more independent. Students can prepare meals independently without assistance.

In culinary school, one of the most rewarding experiences is seeing a student like Jeremy use his creativity. He has gradually tested his creativity and experimented with the recipes in this book over the years. From learning how to make a simple sauce or salad dressing from Chef Rome to creating something decadent and special like dinnertime casseroles, Jeremy has stretched the limits of his palate, imagination, and self-care abilities.

It is also an opportunity for students to learn about different cultures from both their peers and guest chefs while advancing their studies as they learn about international cuisines. When this knowledge is gained by the students, it awakens an open-mindedness within them, and takes them on a journey of new tastes such as when Jeremy first tried couscous and realized it was pasta.

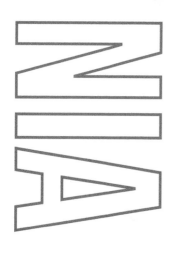

Cooking is an act of self-care, and we are constantly reminding the students that we are all worthy of a home-cooked meal.

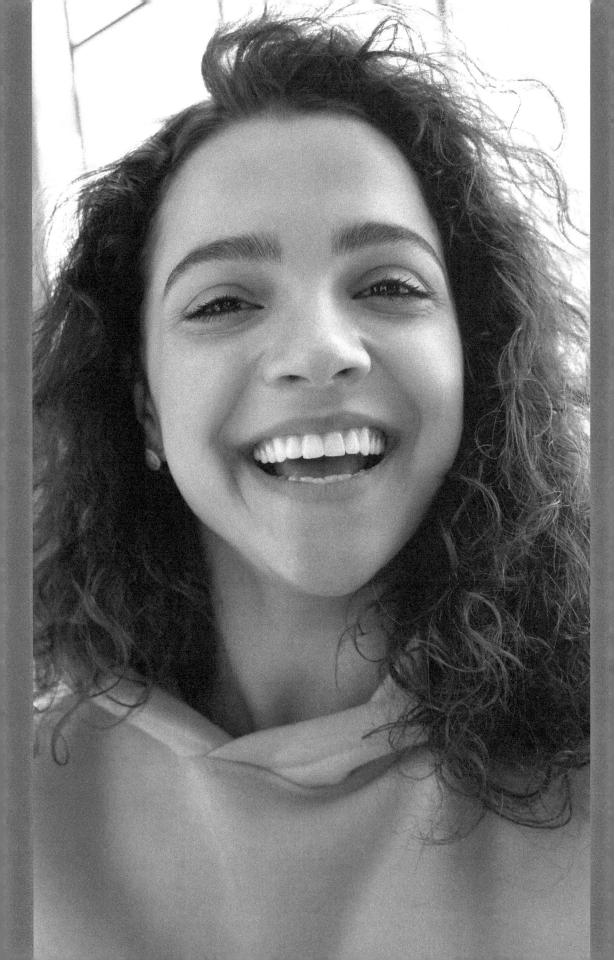

NIA

Baking and cooking can be two very different things depending on the person. The key is to find the right recipe.

Nia, a bright 21-year-old student with autism, says "when the work becomes more complex, it is easier to become overwhelmed." However, some kids who prefer structure may find these complex recipes appealing,

Ms. Zipporah said. "Pick what feels right for you." Ms. Z reminds the class, "If you like something, it must be right." Mindful hobbies can be useful therapy tools. The act of cooking is an act of self-care, and we constantly remind our students that we are all deserving of a homecooked meal. Ms. Z quietly reminds Nia, as she prepares pasta and summer vegetables for lunch, "When you prepare mindfully for your family, they will notice the thoughtfulness and consideration you have put into the meal, and this is how you can take care of others as well as yourself. Be mindful of your work, your steps in the process, your knife skills, and of course the finished product," Ms. Z explains as they go through a mindful cooking method.

As a result of Nia's autism, she can cook well. Because she has a sensory processing disorder, some of Nia's senses work better than others. Nia is instructed by Ms. Z to be mindful of the sounds, smells, textures, and other physical sensations of the kitchen to practice mindfulness. "Before we begin cooking, we all know that we should not have our mobile devices on display. Ms. Z explains that doing too many things at once reduces the effectiveness of the brain. When there are too many things going on at the same time, it becomes difficult for students with diverse learning needs to switch between tasks.

Since becoming a chef, Nia has learned to consciously consider each ingredient she works with. How does it taste, smell, and what is its texture?

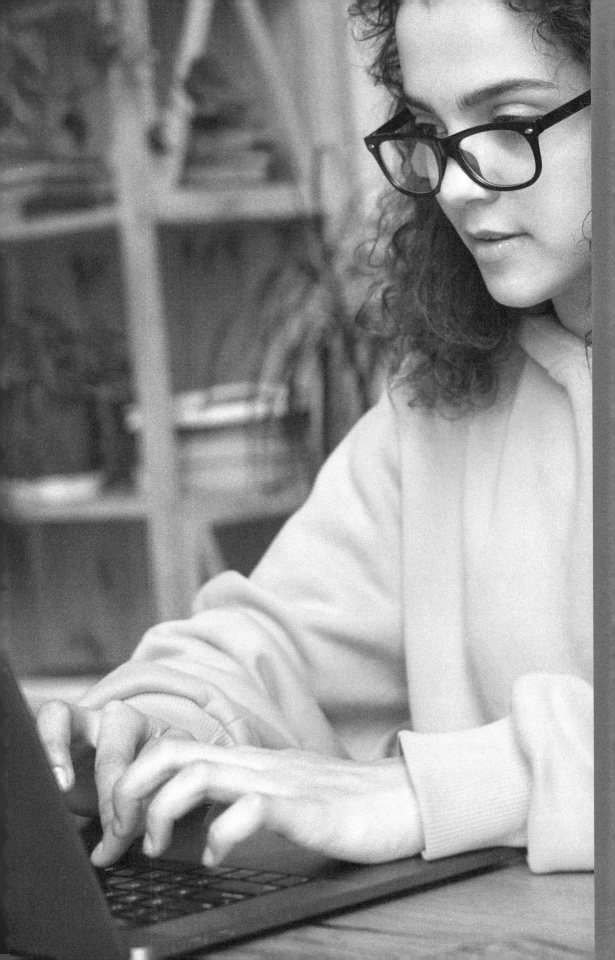

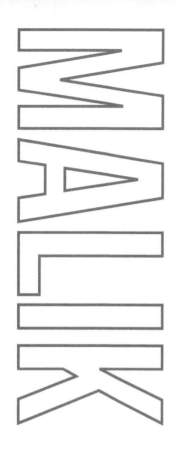

MALIK

Trauma-informed spaces
provide a system of
support.

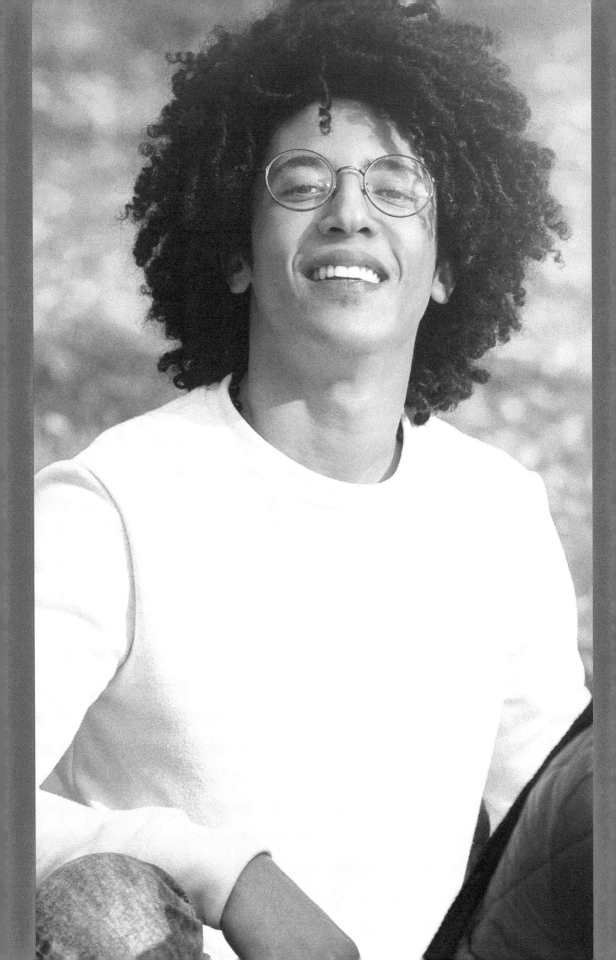

MALIK

In Malik's high school file, there are numerous references to his anger outbursts. His trauma was evident when he came to iCan Dream Center in his sophomore year of high school. Mr. Matt, one of Malik's teachers in our accelerated high school credit recovery program, said, "Human beings do not react with anger in this manner without reason." Mr. Matt began working with Malik in the same way he works with all the young people who come through his door, with a spirit of connection over restriction.

Before we can start structuring that student according to a rule-following model, we must connect, plain and simple. The social worker at the iCan Dream Center showed Malik how to perform a simple repetitive movement exercise. When he was upset, we simply made him tap his finger repeatedly, and you could see the anger leave his body until he was just sitting there breathing calmly. "Do you see what you have just done," a social worker whispered to Malik. Showing him just one small thing he can control restores some peace.

In an all-staff healing circle, Dr. Ford reminds the team that it's becoming increasingly understood that a child's adverse childhood experiences (ACES) can contribute to behaviors such as short attention spans and anger outbursts. "I believe there is a reason behind this, and maybe if we had a little more compassion and understanding about the reason, we may be able to have a better outcome with this child or adult," explains Dr. Ford. "Traditionally, when students have emotional outbursts, the teacher's perspective was that they were being difficult or not paying attention." However, we have been talking about getting to the root of behavior since we were established; our programs were born from this approach.

Every time I hire a staff member, from transportation drivers to teacher aides, to program administrators, I pay particular attention to whether that person demonstrates qualities of empathy and compassion for youth experiencing trauma. Dr. Ford states that sometimes trauma is simply a consequence of years of being labeled the "bad kid." Ford explains, "Previously, we have said what is wrong with the child, or what is wrong with the adult. But now we are saying what has happened?"

Spaces that are trauma-informed provide a system of support. In addition to food insecurity, the culinary program addresses the root causes of the emotional challenges our students and families face. In his culinary group, Malik thrives. Cooking at the program has influenced him profoundly. "I would like to make pizza and pasta and everything else. Maybe I will open Malik's pizzeria," says the jovial teen wearing a hoodie. Students are taught about healthy food, gardening, and composting. "That dirt lies at the bottom of the plant and represents the earth, growth; there is always the possibility of resilience in living things," says Mr. Matt. He hopes that Malik will take some of these lessons with him. "Malik made a large pot of beef vegetable soup. He went home to his house, which did not have electricity, and shared his soup with a neighbor," recalled Mr. Matt. "I feel great just knowing that I can do something like this, I can help my neighbors. That is cool," Malik says with a shy smile.

66 Spaces that are trauma-informed provide a system of support. Sometimes trauma is simply a consequence of years of being labeled the "bad kid." Previously, we have asked 'what is wrong with the child, or what is wrong with the adult.' But now we are saying, 'what happened to you?' **99**

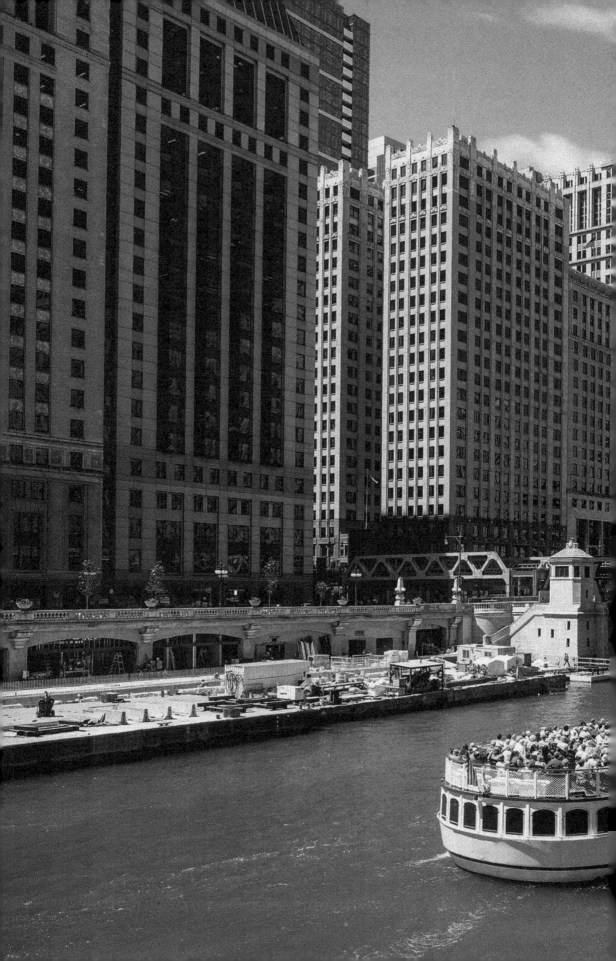

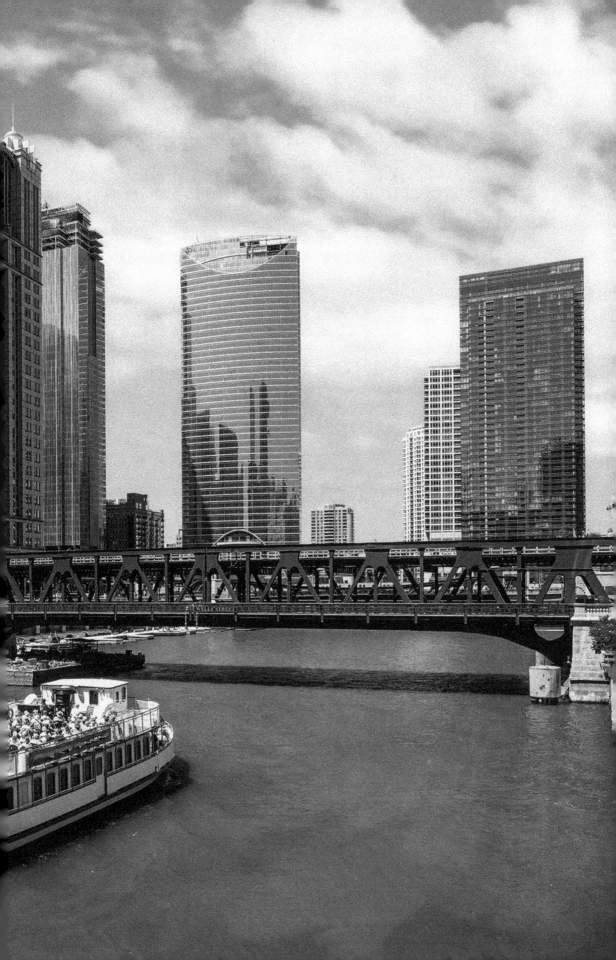

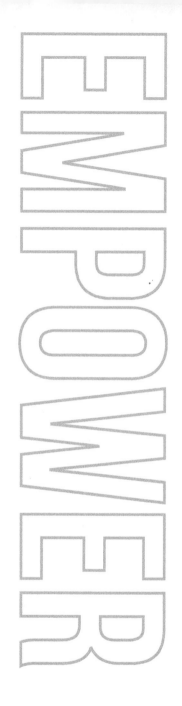

EMPOWER

In the recipes that follow, you'll get a taste of just how empowered our students have been in the kitchen. Enjoy these dishes and know that they are the very expression of the students' originality and creativity.

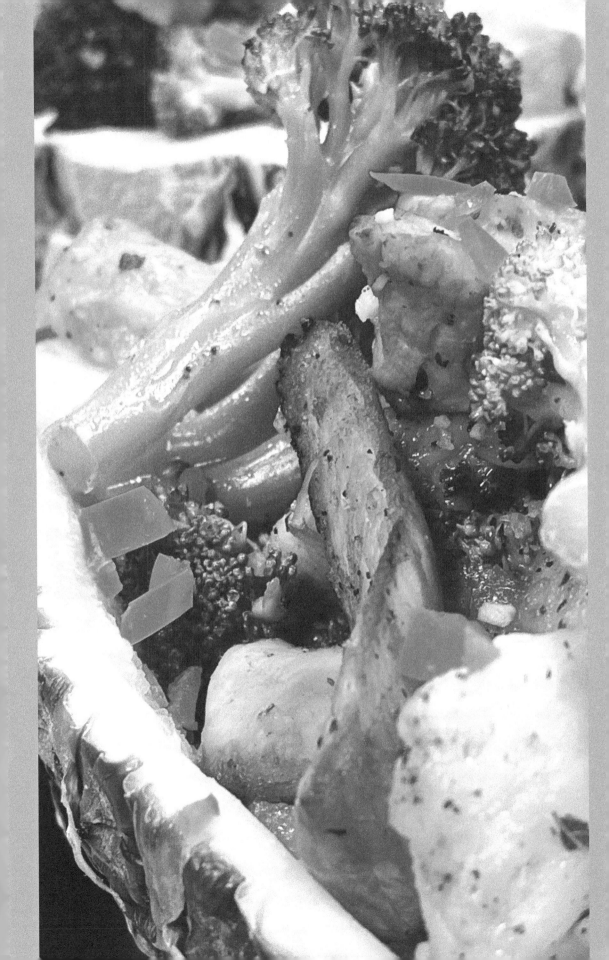

EMPOWER

An outstanding student of ours wrote beautiful prose; Kelly was very kind and helpful to other students in a quiet way; she was also an excellent cook. She did not share any of her skills as a writer or in the kitchen with her teachers in high school.

Kelly, a stunning and intelligent young woman, was suffering from an extreme anxiety disorder because of which she was a selective mute. Despite years of therapy, her voice had not been heard for over a decade, which represented more than half of her life. She enrolled in our postsecondary transition program after graduating from high school. The family was naturally concerned about Kelly's ability to handle adult life despite her remarkable intellect. In the end, they selected iCan Dream Center after visiting several programs, as our second location has a kitchen that serves as a focal point just beyond the reception area. While waiting patiently for me to complete my conversation with several other parents on the program tour, I could almost see the pride in her father's eyes. As I approached him, he spun around on our rainbow-colored bar stool, holding his cellphone in hand. He was eager to show me a video that he had managed to capture of his daughter softly speaking in her favorite place-the kitchen. I was told that Kelly had taken the initiative in preparing meals for the family before she entered high school, including during holidays.

If I could reach through this page and offer you a taste of Kelly's homemade bread, I would not do so for fear that you might bite my hand. Kelly first enrolled in the program in 2017, when culinary arts was used to enhance science instruction, support executive functioning by providing students with an opportunity to plan and prepare for a celebration held at the iCan Dream Center.

As a result of this student, I have a deeper understanding of how cooking can level the playing field for our students. We revised our schedule to include culinary arts as a regular part of the curriculum at that point. As a result, we have included many activities that we believe would EMPOWER our students. We strive to make learning relevant to them. We embrace this type of planning, even though it may appear laborious, because of the positive effect it has on our community.

The voice of Chris, our student who advocated for the establishment of a school choir, was not the only one amplified. Our student Ben, who informed us that he was unable to wash clothes, is one of many who gain more than just life skills when we visit the laundromat. Well, guess what? Kelly was not the only one whose voice was most easily heard in the kitchen.

Throughout the recipes that follow, you will gain a sense of just how accomplished our students have been in the kitchen. Take pleasure in these dishes and keep in mind that they are the expression of the student's creativity and originality.

66 We have incorporated many activities that we know would EMPOWER our students. This student deepened my mindset around how cooking can level the playing field for our students. 99

DEE DEE'S
BBQ MEATBALLS

Serves: 10

INGREDIENTS

3 Pounds of ground chuck

1 Yellow onion *(fine chopped)*

1 Tablespoon of seasoned salt

½ Tablespoon of ground pepper

½ Tablespoon of onion powder

½ Tablespoon of garlic powder

2oz. Ice cream scoop

3 Bottles of your favorite barbecue sauce *(1 pound bottles)*

½ Cup of lite brown sugar

½ Cup of orange juice

1 Crock Pot

DIRECTIONS

In a large bowl, combine the ground beef with half the fine chopped onions, seasoned salt, pepper, onion powder, and garlic powder. Mix well. Place a large skillet onto the stove on medium high. Use the ice cream scoop to portion out the meatballs. Add the meatballs to the skillet. Brown the meatballs on all sides. Drain the excess grease from the skillet and repeat until all the meatballs have been browned. Transfer the meatballs to the crockpot. Turn the crockpot on medium. Add to the skillet the bbq sauce, brown sugar and orange juice. Bring to a simmer and cook for about 10 minutes. Pour the bbq sauce and remaining onions over the meatballs. Cover and let cook for about an hour. Serve hot!

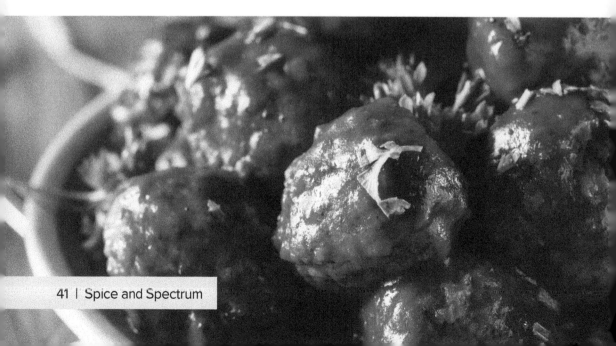

ZIPPORAH'S EASY-GOING PEACH COBBLER

Serves: 10

INGREDIENTS

2 Cans of sliced peaches in heavy syrup *(13 ounce cans)*

1 Tablespoon of vanilla extract

1 Cup of white sugar

½ Cup of lite brown sugar

2 Teaspoons of ground nutmeg

1 ½ Sticks of salted butter

2 Cans of croissant dough

Casserole dish

DIRECTIONS

Pre-heat the oven to 350. In a large sauce pot, pour in the peaches, vanilla, sugars, nutmeg and 1 stick of butter. Allow the sauce to come to a boil. Once the sauce has reached the boiling temperature, reduce to simmer. Cook for about 30 minutes.

Slice the remaining half stick of butter and place into the casserole dish. Place the dish into the oven until melted. Remove from the oven and place onto the stove. Use a paper towel to spread the butter all over the dish.

Turn off the stove and spoon the peaches into the casserole dish. Spread evenly. Top the peaches with the croissant dough. Press the dough down into the syrup with a spoon while placing some peaches on top of the dough.

Place into the oven and bake for 25-30 minutes or until the crust is golden brown. Remove from the oven and let it cool. Enjoy!

" Everything is peachy queen "

APPLE FRIES

Serves: 4

INGREDIENTS

3 Apples *(red or golden delicious)* *(cut into French fries)*

2 Cups of water

Juice of 1 lemon

½ Cup of corn starch

2 Cups of vegetable oil

DIRECTIONS

Place a large skillet onto the stove on medium high. Allow the oil to heat up to about 375. Use a thermometer to see the temperature.

In a large bowl, combine the apples, water and lemon juice. Mix well. This will keep the apples from turning brown.

Allow the apples to sit in the lemon water for about 5 minutes. Drain well for about 5 minutes. Sprinkle the corn starch over the apples. Use more corn starch if necessary to ensure the apples are well coated.

While using a slotted spoon, carefully place the apples in the oil. Let the apples cook for about 4 minutes or until golden brown. Remove the fries from the oil and place onto a paper towel lined platter or plate. Drain well. Sprinkle the fries with a pinch of cinnamon and sugar. Enjoy this quick, simple and easy snack.

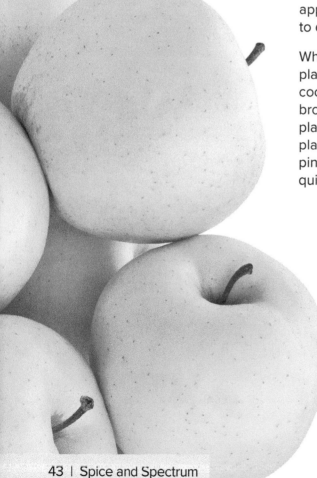

66 Taste the
tart crunch 99

PINEAPPLE CHICKEN & BROCCOLI

Serves: 4

INGREDIENTS

4 Boneless skinless chicken breast halves *(cut into bite size pieces)*

½ Cup of all-purpose flour

1 Teaspoon of salt or seasoned salt

1 Teaspoon of black pepper

2 Tablespoons of olive oil

½ Cup of diced pineapple

3 Quarters of a cup of broccoli crowns

½ Cup of pineapple juice

DIRECTIONS

Place a large skillet onto the stove on medium high. Rinse the chicken under cold water, then pat dry with a paper towel. Set aside.

In a small mixing bowl, combine the flour, salt, and pepper. Mix well. Add the oil to the skillet. Place the chicken into the flour mixture. Shake off the extra flour and carefully place the chicken into the skillet. Cook for about 3 minutes on each side. Add the pineapple, broccoli and pineapple juice. Cover with a lid. Reduce the heat to medium low. Continue to cook for about 4 minutes. Remove the chicken from the skillet and place onto the plate. Spoon the pineapple and broccoli over the chicken and enjoy with your favorite rice or pasta.

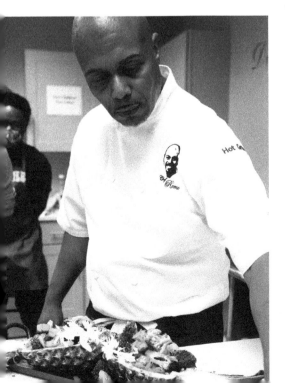

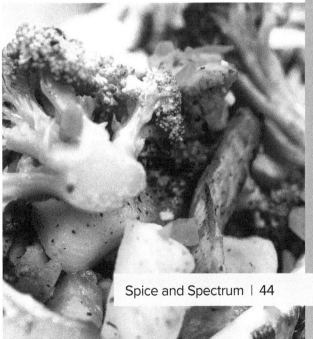

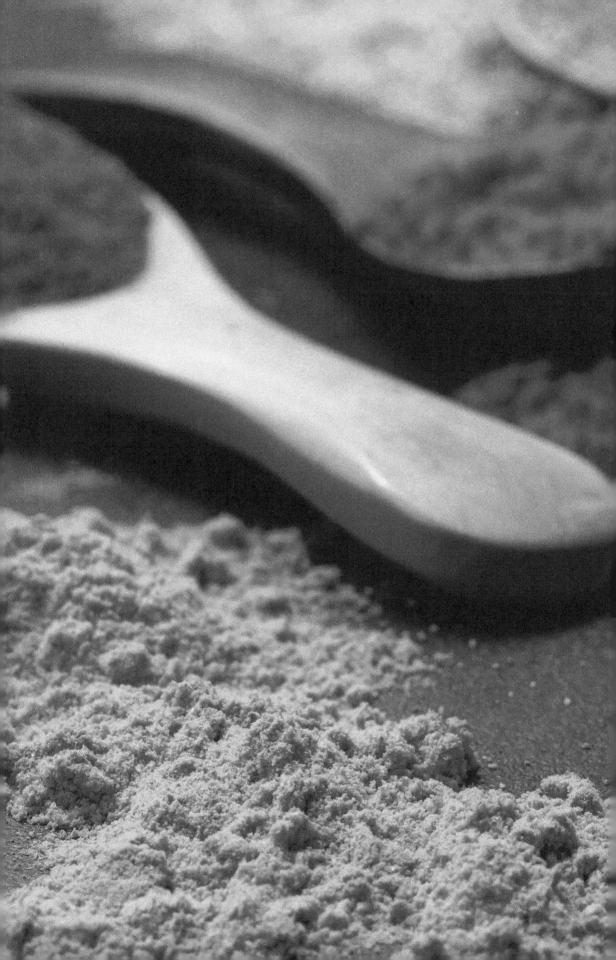

THE 'I CAN DREAM' TANGERINE JERK VINAIGRETTE

Serves: 10

INGREDIENTS

1 Shallot *(chopped)*

1 Tablespoon of vegetable oil

½ Bottle of white wine vinegar

¼ Cup of sugar

5 Tangerines *(Freshly squeezed)* *(save the peels)*

Pinch of salt

1 Tablespoon of dry Smokey rub

½ Tablespoon of mild jerk seasoning

¼ Cup of lite olive oil

DIRECTIONS

Place a large skillet onto the stove on medium high. Allow the pan to heat up for about 4 minutes. In the meantime, chop the shallot and add it to the pan. Add the oil. Sauté the shallot for about 4 minutes. Pour in the vinegar and reduce the heat to medium. Cook for about 5 minutes Add the sugar and stir until the sugar dissolves. Add the tangerines and the peels. Continue to cook for about 10 minutes. Add the remaining ingredients. Mix well. Remove from the stove and pour the vinaigrette into a small bowl. Once the vinaigrette is cool, adjust the flavor by adding more vinegar or sugar or sugar if desired.

Toss with your favorite salad greens. I recommend arugula.

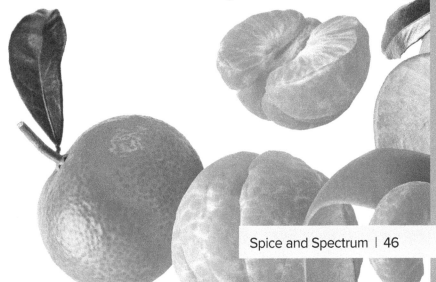

RASPBERRY CHICKEN

Serves: 4

INGREDIENTS

4 Boneless skinless chicken breasts

½ Cup of all-purpose flour

1 Teaspoon of salt

1 Teaspoon of pepper

¼ Cup of olive oil

2 Tablespoons of unsalted butter

1 Teaspoon of dry tarragon

½ Cup of frozen raspberries

½ Cup of chicken broth

DIRECTIONS

Place a large skillet on the stove on medium high. Wash the chicken under cold water and set aside. In a mixing bowl, combine the flour, salt, and pepper. Mix well.

Place the oil into the skillet. Coat the chicken in the flour mixture. Shake off the excess flour and place the breast into the skillet. Sauté the chicken for three minutes on each side. Add the tarragon leaves, raspberries and chicken broth. Reduce the heat to medium low. Let the breast simmer for about 10 minutes or until the sauce thickens. Serve over rice.

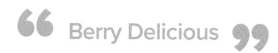 **Berry Delicious**

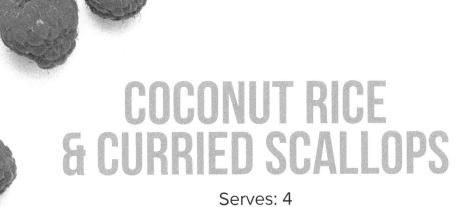

COCONUT RICE
& CURRIED SCALLOPS

Serves: 4

INGREDIENTS

2 Cups of jasmine rice

1 ½ Cups of water

2 Cans of unsweetened coconut milk *(use 1 cup for the rice, reserve the rest for later use)*

1 Tablespoon of butter *(salted)*

1 Tablespoon of vegetable oil

12 Large sea scallops *(size U10)*

2 Teaspoons of curry powder

1 Shallot *(chopped)*

1 Roma tomato *(chopped)*

1 Teaspoon of minced garlic

1 Teaspoon of ground turmeric

2 Cups of baby spinach

DIRECTIONS

Rinse the rice under cold water and drain. Place a sauce pot onto the stove. Pour in the rice, water, 1 cup of coconut milk. Bring to a boil. Cover with a tight-fitting lid and reduce the heat to the lowest setting. Cook for about 12 – 15 minutes. Remove the rice from the stove and set aside.

In the meantime, place a skillet onto the stove on medium high. Add the butter and oil to the skillet. Once the oil is hot, add the scallops. Cook the scallops for about 2 minutes on each side. Remove the scallops to the side for a moment. Reduce the heat to medium low. Add to the pan the curry powder, shallots, garlic, turmeric. Add the remaining coconut milk. Let the sauce simmer for about 5 minutes on low. Add the spinach to the skillet and return the scallops to the pan as well.

Place the rice in the center of the plate. Arrange the scallops around the rice. Spoon the sauce over the scallops and enjoy.

SWEET POTATO CORN MUFFINS

Serves: 8

INGREDIENTS

SWEET POTATO RECIPE

1 Large sweet potato *(peel and dice into bite size pieces)*

1 Teaspoon of nutmeg
(freshly ground is best)

1 Teaspoon of ground cinnamon

½ Stick of salted butter

½ Tablespoon of vanilla extract

¼ Cup of orange juice

1 Tablespoon of lite brown sugar

1 Tablespoon of sugar

CORN MUFFIN MIX

1 Cup of yellow cornmeal

1 Tablespoon of baking powder

½ Cup of sugar

Pinch of salt

1 ¼ Cups of milk

1/3 Cup of vegetable oil

2 Large eggs *(beaten)*

DIRECTIONS

SWEET POTATO RECIPE

Place a 2–3-quart pot onto the stove on medium high. Combine all the ingredients in the pot. Cover with a tight-fitting lid or foil. Cook for about 20 – 25 minutes. Once the sweet potato is fork tender, turn off the stove. Whip until the potatoes are smooth like mashed potatoes. Set aside for later use.

CORN MUFFIN MIX

Pre-heat the oven to 375. In a mixing bowl, combine all the ingredients and mix well. Add the sweet potato mixture into the muffin mix. Mix well. Spoon the mixture into a lightly greased muffin pan. Fill about ¾ full. Let the mixture sit for about 5 minutes before placing the pan into the oven.

Cook for about 20 minutes. Once the muffins are done, remove them from the oven and allow to cool for about 5 minutes. Enjoy!

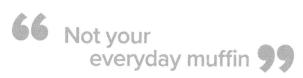 " Not your everyday muffin "

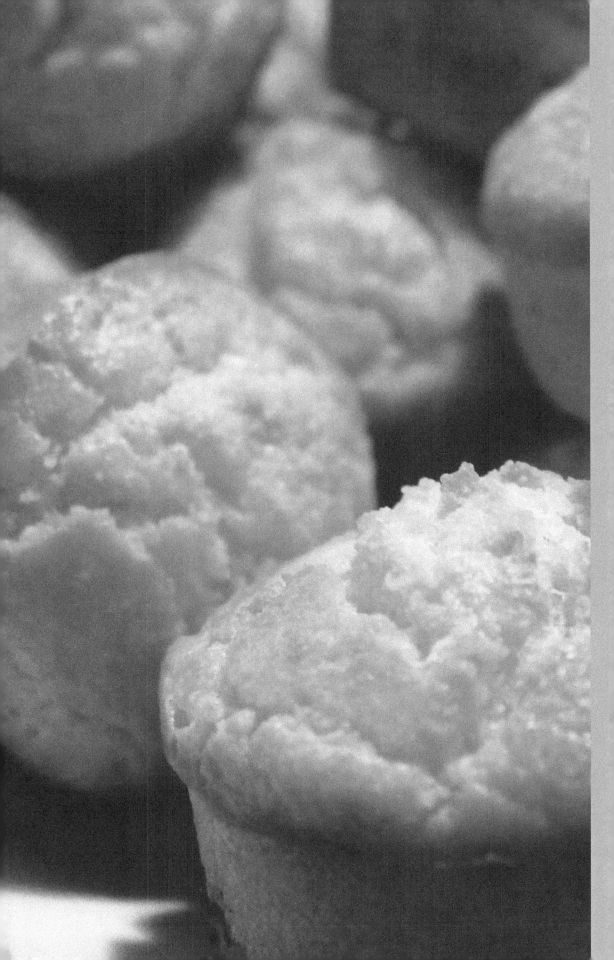

THE BEST BAKED BEANS

Serves: 10

INGREDIENTS

1 Pound of ground beef or ground turkey

1 Small yellow onion *(chopped)*

1 Green bell pepper *(chopped)*

1 Teaspoon of crushed red pepper flakes

2 Pounds of can pork and beans

¼ Cup of brown sugar

¼ Cup of white sugar

1 Tablespoon of ground cinnamon

1 Tablespoon of yellow mustard

2 Tablespoon of vanilla extract

1/3 Cup of BBQ sauce

DIRECTIONS

Pre-heat the oven to 350. Place a skillet on the stove on medium high. Add the ground meat, onion, and bell pepper. Brown the meat until done. Drain the majority of the grease. Add the remaining ingredients in a casserole dish and mix well. Cover with foil and place into the oven. Cook for one hour. Remove from the oven and carefully remove the foil. Enjoy!

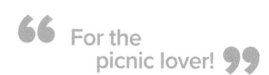 For the picnic lover!

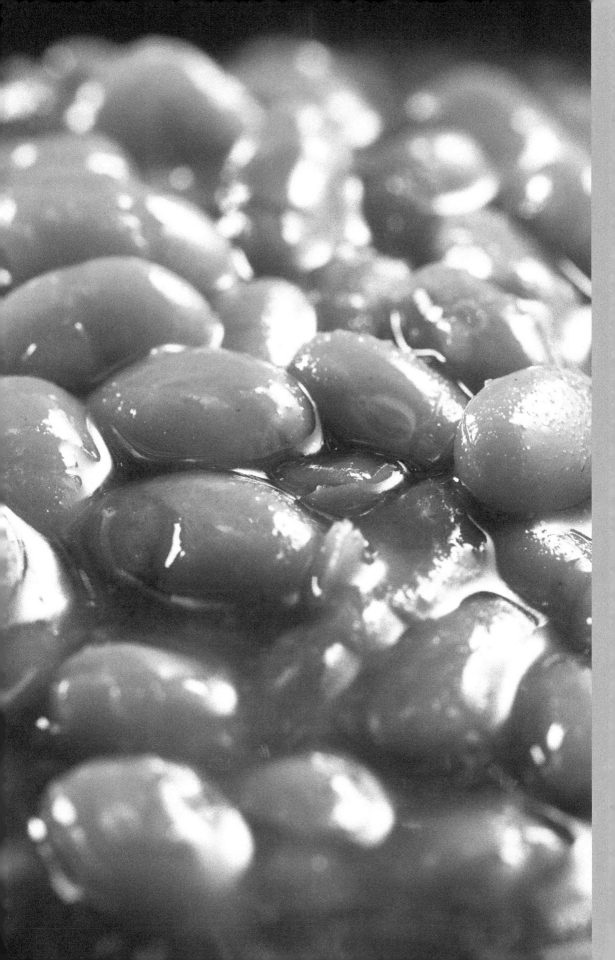

HAMBURGER YAKISOBA

Serves: 8

INGREDIENTS

1 Box of spaghetti noodles

Salt

Olive oil

1 Pound of lean ground beef or ground turkey

1 Small red bell pepper

1 Small green bell pepper

2 Stalks of celery *(thin sliced at an angle)*

3 Green onions *(chopped)*

1 Teaspoon of cayenne pepper

¼ Cup of Worcestershire sauce

¼ Cup of low sodium soy sauce

2 Teaspoons of garlic powder

DIRECTIONS

Place a 5 quart pot onto the stove on high. Bring the water to a boil. Add the salt, olive oil, and spaghetti. Use a pasta spoon and mix well for about one minute to prevent the pasta from sticking. Cook the pasta according to the directions on the box.

In the meantime, place a large skillet onto the stove on medium high. Place the ground meat, bell peppers, celery, and green onions into the skillet and cook until the meat has browned. If there's a lot of grease, drain about half of it off.

Once the pasta is cooked, drain well and rinse under hot water. Add the remaining ingredients and mix well. Combine the pasta with the meat and toss well until the meat is evenly distributed. Enjoy!

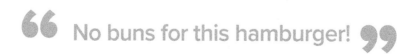

66 No buns for this hamburger! **99**

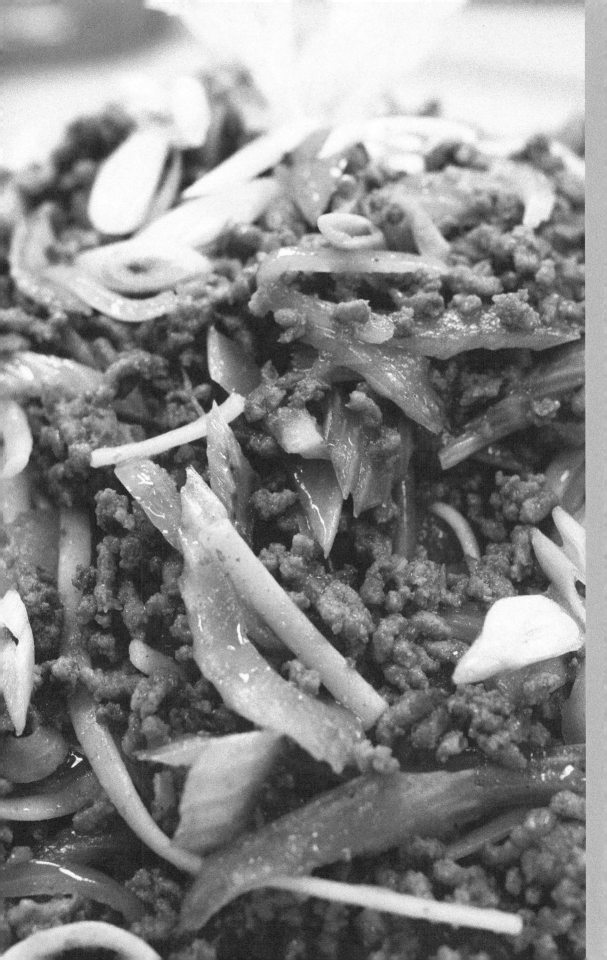

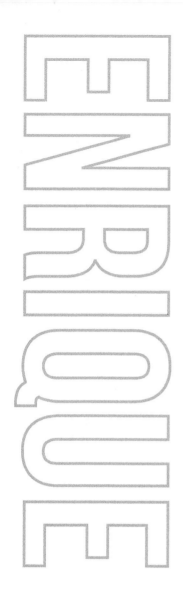

ENRIQUE

Studies show that the intersection of food and family can have a positive impact on mental health.

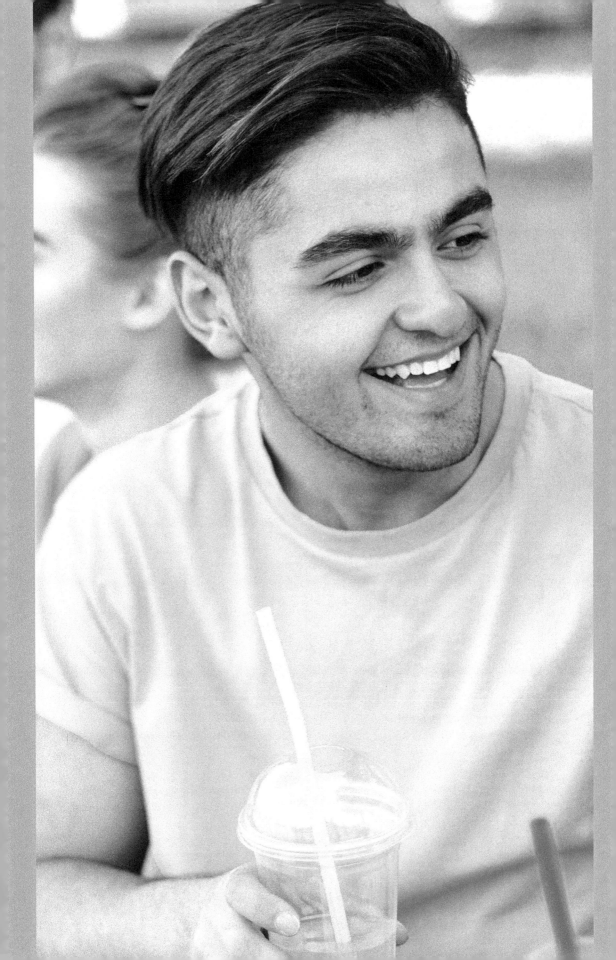

ENRIQUE

When Enrique first came to iCan Dream Center as a tenth grader, he told us he did not feel smart. What's most important about that statement is that nearly all our students have gone through school internalizing a similar feeling—that they are not smart enough for the worlds they inhabit in school.

When we got down to the root cause of why Enrique did not feel smart, he talked about being a younger student and knowing he did not belong at the table with the kids who could already read. He described what we knew to be a common experience students report having felt early in their educational careers—the years when they felt their first loss of control as a student. Enrique admitted to being out of control for a period in his young life as a teenager. "I am pretty much out of control a lot and don't have any control over my emotions. It's more that I have anxiety attacks over certain things."

As we began to work with Enrique, he became soothed that the feeling of being out of control was natural. The generalized educational setting can be a stressful place for students with learning disabilities of all stripes, and the stress only ramps up without very targeted interventions and supports early on. The realization that Enrique needed some locus of control led to a turning point where Enrique was able to begin to dream about what might come next for him after high school.

Working with a social worker and in peer groups helped Enrique self-actualize, which is so important for youth. In the high school credit recovery classroom, we work with students like Enrique everyday who struggle to find success in traditional high schools. Some students come to us with only a few credits to their name, others were disengaged during the pandemic and come out of a growing need to recover credits in a smaller, trauma-informed space. In culinary class, students take ownership over their process.

There's a rhythm to the class, but there aren't bells and tests looming, and that makes all the difference in a student leaning into learning. Before coming to iCan Dream Center, Enrique struggled with self-esteem so much that impaired concentration and focus were such a barrier to learning that he was close to dropping out. But, today, he has a sense of agency over his path. He has some input around when to complete an assignment, and most importantly, he enjoys a sense of true connection with his instructors and related service providers and that has been so meaningful.

Connecting with adults is so underrated in teens and young adults and that sense of connection has helped Enrique love himself. As he grows in self-confidence, an emerging desire to plan for what comes next takes seed. Maybe college is not part of the path forward for Enrique, and that is just fine. For now, Enrique thinks he might like to sell cars for a living. As part of his curriculum planning, instructors build coursework that will be useful to move him closer to his goal. Soft skills like relationship-building, decorum, organization, and planning all become important goals. Math skills are refined. Writing solid emails is going to be important, so we work on the skill internally giving him the task of communicating frequently with his instructors in a business email format.

Enrique came to iCan Dream Center not feeling smart. To some, that's not a major life setback. But, just imagine going through life believing that statement and feeling that there is no place for you in the world of school and work. Whether it is in our kitchen or in our classrooms, our students are empowered toward discovering their greatness. Leaving the iCan Dream Center knowing that they ARE smart is just like having climbed their own Mt. Everest. For so many years, people and systems left students like Enrique feeling that he didn't belong. We all deserve a place to belong, dream, and achieve. Enrique is going to sell a lot of cars after high school. We know it. He belongs.

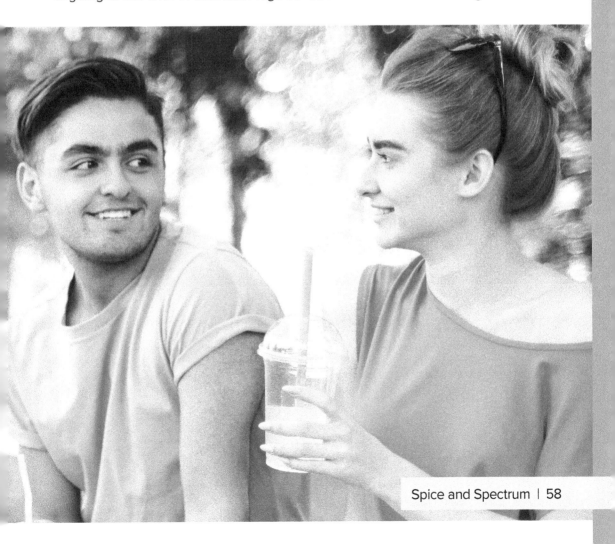

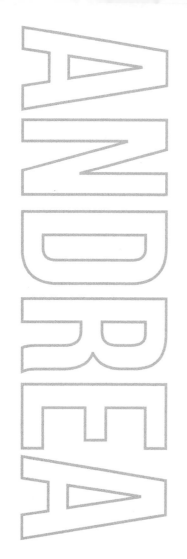

ANDREA

Typical learners emerge into adulthood largely due to circumstance, upbringing, and a gradual uncovering of passion. But for neurodiverse learners, there is often a sea of uncertainties that surround our students' lives.

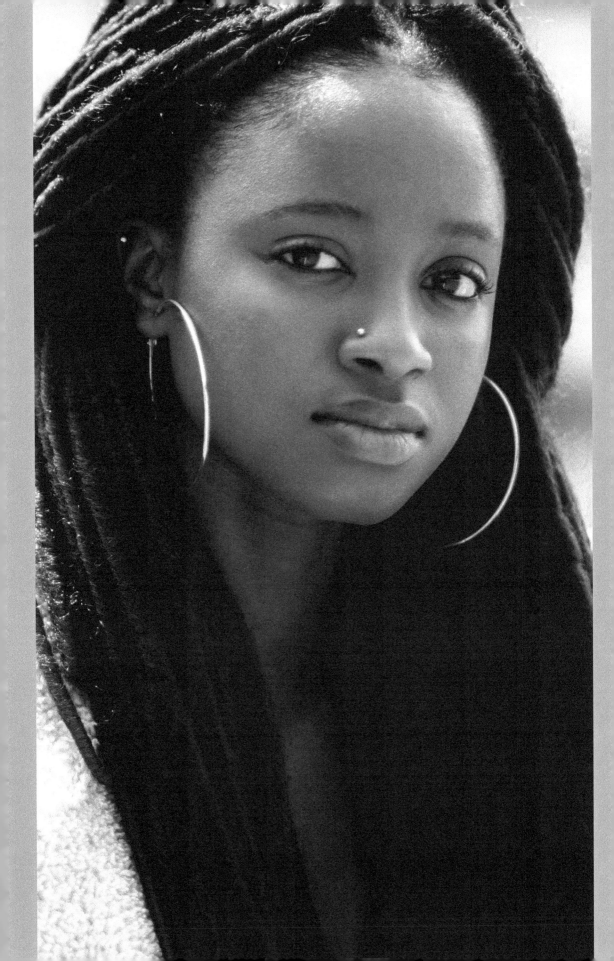

ANDREA

Andrea, an 18-year-old student who enjoys music and shopping, was referred to iCan Dream Center by the social worker at her high school. Andrea has a hard time dealing with criticism. The eleventh grader's school counselor described her as overly reactive to criticism. Andrea is a sensitive, shy, funny teenager who has long had difficulty reading and writing but thrives at iCan Dream Center.

Once we discovered Drea's traumatic childhood, as the daughter of an addicted mother and an absent father, we immediately started to provide her trauma-informed treatment. She spends some of that time in the kitchen with her behavior therapist, Ms. Zipporah. The focus and direction provided by following a recipe is extremely helpful to her. She can anticipate what to expect at every stage. The event that occurs between an adolescent and a bowl of salad greens is not a cataclysmic one, and cooking is therapeutic in that regard.

We speak with the students one-on-one, investigating their difficulties and the reasons behind them, but we also work with students on a cooking project to address academic gaps as well as self-care. From soups, to muffins, waffles, and comfort foods of every kind, cooking empowers the students to find the courage to succeed.

As people grow into adulthood, they are primarily influenced by their circumstances, upbringing, and an awakening of their passion. But for neurodiverse learners, there are often many uncertainties surrounding their lives. Our learners are faced with a lot of challenges in their lives, and we hope that providing them with good nutrition and empowering them with the knowledge and skills to nourish and care for others will have a positive impact on their lives.

While a student's trauma will never be erased by culinary arts, we have found that busying students for an hour in the kitchen has a healing effect. This fortunate reality that we are a family during these hours that we are at the Center together, the unspoken assurance that we will continue to cook peach cobblers together in this small, but mighty kitchen of ours, is often enough for us. We are fortunate in ways that we cannot describe as we wonder about the alternatives for our students.

To prepare the stuffed shells, Drea sets the oven to high heat, and a pan of pasta loaded up with spinach and cheese sits on the counter. A bowl of salad prepared by Drea is waiting, topped with a tangy dill dressing that she and her friends made moments ago. Dessert will consist of brownies and ice cream with fresh raspberries atop. As a result, while a plate full of honest food shared with excellent friends may not be able to erase the past, the sharing of meals with friends can provide the healing we all deserve in the present. Teachers look forward to enjoying every bite and every laugh with these young people who deal with adversities some can never even begin to comprehend.

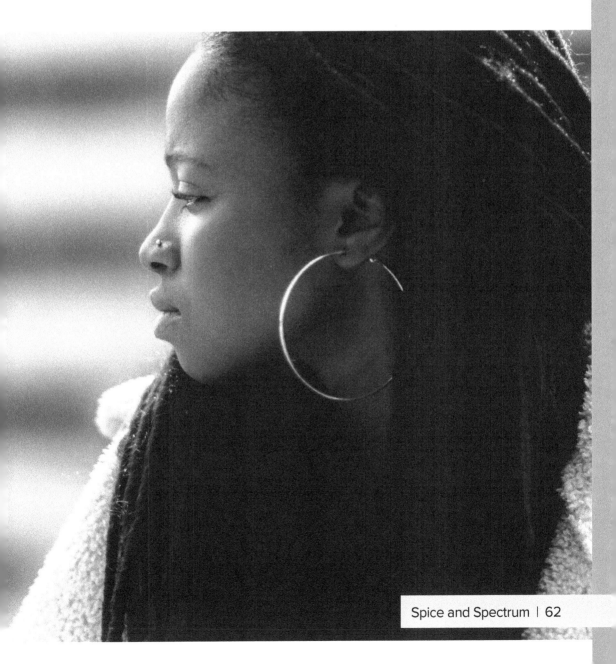

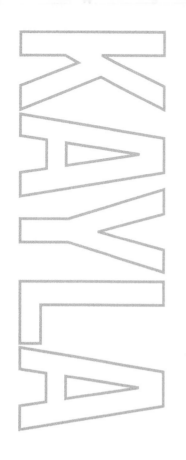

KAYLA

Sometimes love shows up as a piping hot bowl full of mashed potatoes with a river of butter running through it.

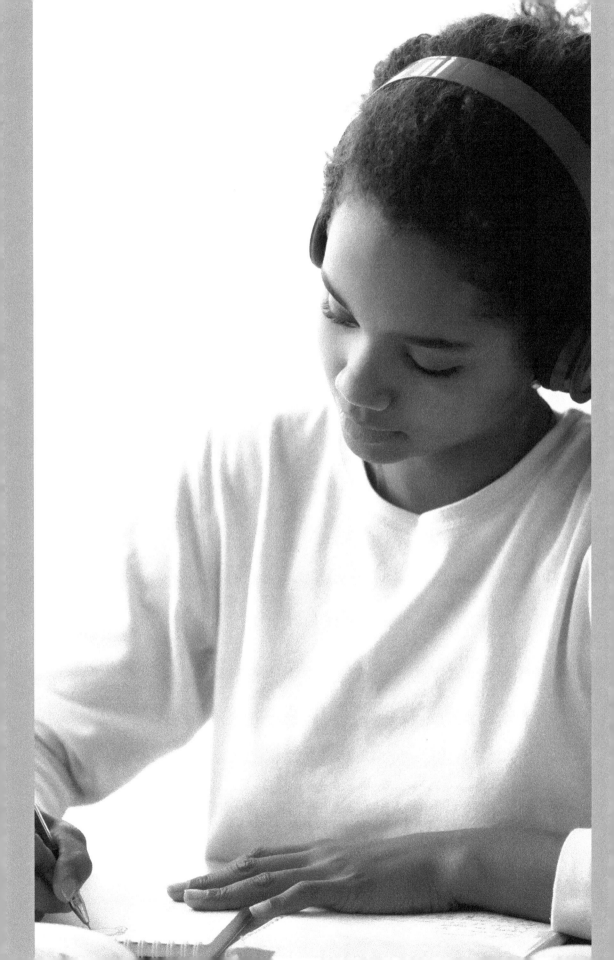

KAYLA

In order to become an accomplished cook one must focus, plan, and pay attention to detail. Our students are striving to improve their knowledge of science, the arts, and math in addition to critical thinking and problem-solving skills.

As a 19-year-old bubbly individual, Kayla works hard on building academic skills that will benefit her in her professional career. Her experience with cooking at iCan Dream has provided her with a background for generalizing her skills. Moreover, the kitchen provides her with the opportunity to practice social skills, or to bond with her friends over bowls of macaroni and cheese or slices of Oreo chocolate cake. In the Dream Café, Kayla and her friends gathered around a long table after attending restorative justice healing circles, financial literacy, and resume writing lessons. As the girls reflect on their mornings, they speak about their families and lament about their relationship difficulties. Kayla demonstrates her emergence as a mature young woman by suggesting that a friend make an appointment to see a therapist about her growing anxiety over a complex family matter. They are looking relaxed and calm at the table; their conversation is natural and unapologetically feminine. As Kayla shares, her mother works long hours; she is tired at the end of the day and often does not have the energy to cook dinner after a double shift. Therefore, her mother frequently brings home mozzarella sticks or pizza.

During the pandemic, Kayla recalls her mother spending days in the kitchen preparing the holiday feast. The family is served turkey, ham, greens, chicken, macaroni, dressing, beans, cornbread, black eyed peas, and one of her mother's infamous cakes. Whether it's red velvet cake, chocolate cake, strawberry shortcake, or caramel crunch, one is better than the next. As Kayla's aunt passed away from COVID-19 complications, her mother took on the role of holiday hostess. In the family room her mom placed her sister's urn and Kayla says her aunt's presence is a comfort to her as the family eats pizza on

Monday night or enjoys a feast on Easter Sunday. Kayla's aunt babysat for her mother when she was very young for her mother to work. Kayla recalls fondly having grown up in a peaceful home where food was always on the table, where children played on the sidewalk in front of the house, and where homemade mashed potatoes were staples for lunches. During the holidays, auntie prepared the family feast. Reminiscing about her childhood, Kayla recalls the little baby sausages and gooey mostaccioli. Seeing a bible verse on the wall reminds the family of the mystery of God's love, love expressed in the form of a piping hot bowl laden with mashed potatoes and a river of butter.

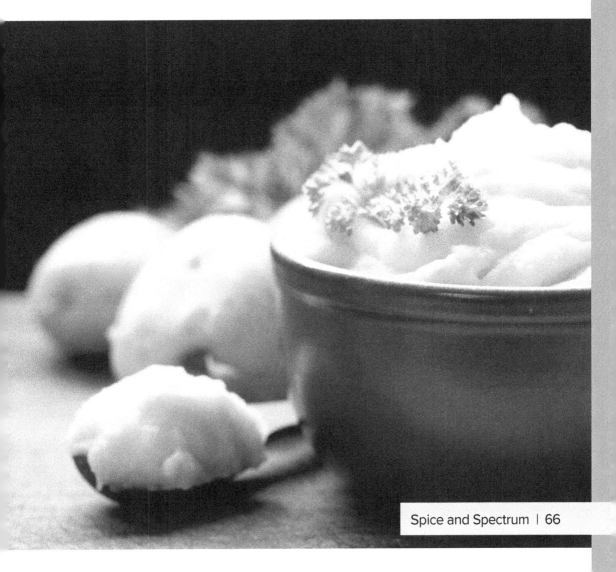

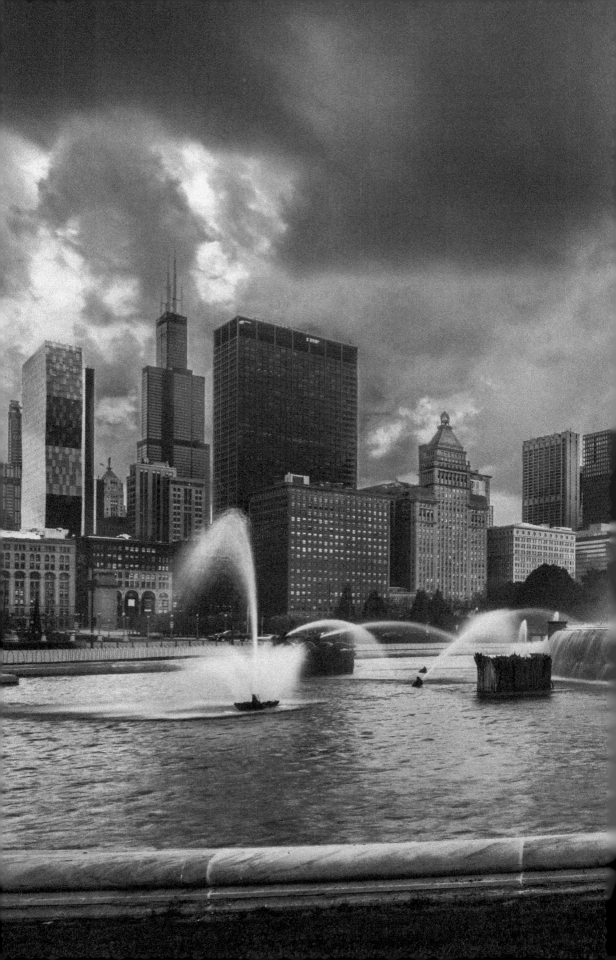

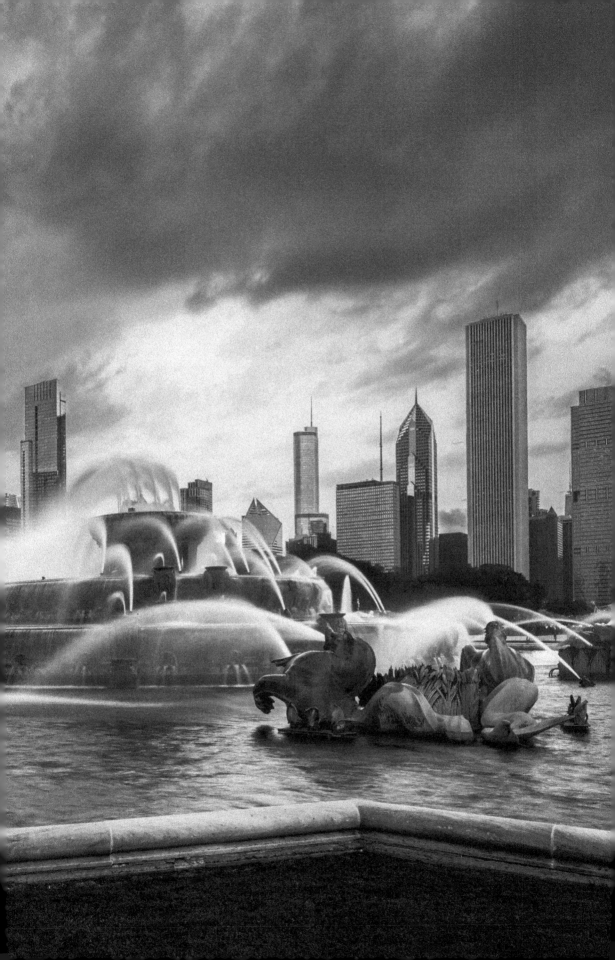

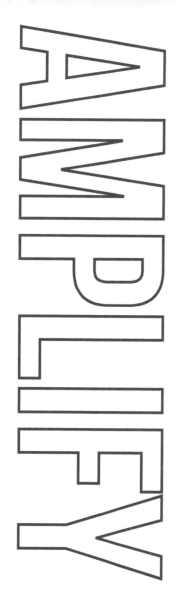

Mexican Pork Chops

The Ultimate Lamb Slider

BBQ Beef Ribs

Jollof Rice

Southern Baked Chicken

BBQ Short Ribs

Linguini with Tomato and Basil Sauce

Skillet Baked Chicken and Salsa

Stovetop Steak

Roasted Cajun Corn

Smothered Liver and Spinach

Baked Chicken and Rice Casserole

Potato Leek and Crab Soup

Apple Glazed Pork Tenderloin

Oxtail Ragu over Pappardelle Pasta

Korean Beef and Brown Rice

Sweet Thai Snapper

Pistachio Crusted Lamb Chop Finished
with a Wild Blueberry Sauce

Savory Beef and Noodles

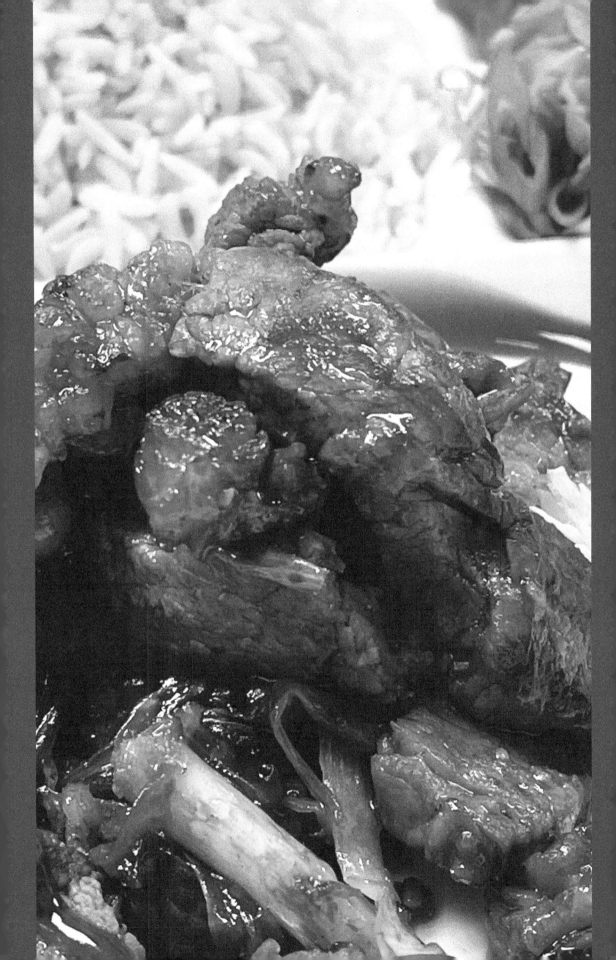

AMPLIFY

During the opening of our 4,000 square foot location, we had a huge commercial coffee machine that occupied nearly all of the counter space in our kitchen. I agreed to this because I love coffee and wanted to make that offering available to our guests. It turns out that many of our parents liked coffee as well.

Our doors opened during the summer, but as Chicago's colder weather began to set in, we noticed a greater interest in our hot drink. Additionally, our enrollment increased! We were paying more for our commercial lease than my monthly mortgage payment at the time, which was quite intimidating. In the early days of this grassroots initiative, multiple roles outside of iCan Dream Center were filled to generate income to support this cause. It would take years for me to feel comfortable putting myself on the payroll. My attention is drawn to this because I was compensated in a different way, and it brought great joy to my heart to engage in coffee chats with others. Consequently, requests for coffee increased with the increasing student enrollment. Our pick-up time was extended from 6pm to 6:45pm to provide parents with a space to arrive, have a seat, decompress from the day, and then begin the responsibility of being a parent.

Being a parent is a challenging and emotional task for anyone seeking to fulfill the role. Parenting a child with a disability represents the "typical" demand multiplied by ten. The families spoke of their relief in having iCan Dream Center create a recreational area for their teens in which they would be regarded as emerging adults while acknowledging their disabilities. There were stories shared by parents about how they managed to juggle appointments for therapy and doctor visits with meetings for IEPs and other school-related activities.

A child with disabilities puts a great deal of burden on the family and marriage, as I knew from my research. Parents of disabled children experience a higher rate of divorce than parents whose children develop normally. I was astonished to hear parents describe the way their grief, regret, blame, and exhaustion were brought to the forefront in their daily lives. Seeing the community that was built around sharing parenting experiences, vulnerability, and cups of coffee was truly gratifying, inspiring, and empowering.

I recall one parent recounting how when she learned that she would have a child with a disability, she did not inform her husband. Her emotions are marked by shame and fear that he will leave the marriage because of this.

Throughout her pregnancy, she carried both her incredible child and the weight of her fears completely alone. As I listened, the hair at the back of my neck stood at attention. Upon reflecting on my own journey as a parent, I recall the intoxicating joy I experienced as I awaited the birth of my son and came to realize how privileged I was. Because of this privilege, I AMPLIFY the cause. iCan Dream Center has developed or incorporated programs based on pain points expressed by parents. Our culinary arts program is no exception.

Parents of children enrolled in our after-school program told us that they wish to see their children develop independence. We initiated a weekly "foods" activity for our students which required an extraordinary amount of creativity as our first location did not include a stove or oven! Looking back, we find our early food activities humorous. Despite the lack of a stove, we went to great lengths to ensure that the cooking activities were engaging and meaningful. One constant has been the level of creativity, care, and attentiveness to the needs of the families we serve.

We have invited iCan Dream families to share their favorite recipes in this section of the cookbook. If this book were a house, the following pages would represent the living room.

66 Every program that we have developed or incorporated at iCan Dream Center was based upon a pain point expressed by a parent. The culinary arts program is no different. **99**

MEXICAN PORK CHOPS

Serves: 6

INGREDIENTS

6 Center cup bone in pork chops

1 Cup of all-purpose flour

1 Cup of vegetable oil

1 Tablespoon of cumin

1 Tablespoon of smoked paprika

½ Tablespoon of garlic powder

1 Teaspoon of black pepper

1 Tablespoon of seasoned salt

1 Cup of chicken broth

1 Can of fire roasted tomatoes

1 Jalapeño *(seeds removed, chopped)*

Juice of 1 lime

1 Tablespoon of chopped cilantro

DIRECTIONS

Place a large skillet on the stove on medium high. Add the oil to the skillet. In a large bowl, combine the flour and spices. Mix well. Coat the chops in the flour. Shake off the excess flour and carefully place the chops in the oil. Allow the chops to cook for about 4 minutes on each side. Add the remaining ingredients. Cover the skillet with a lid or foil. Reduce the heat to simmer for about 30 minutes. Serve with your favorite rice or pasta.

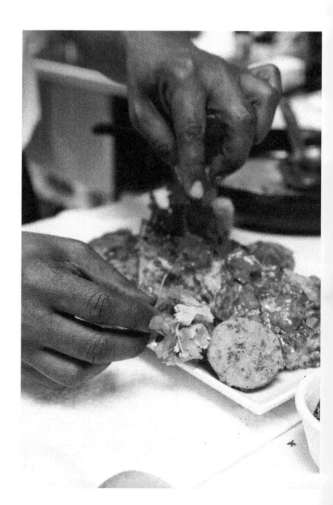

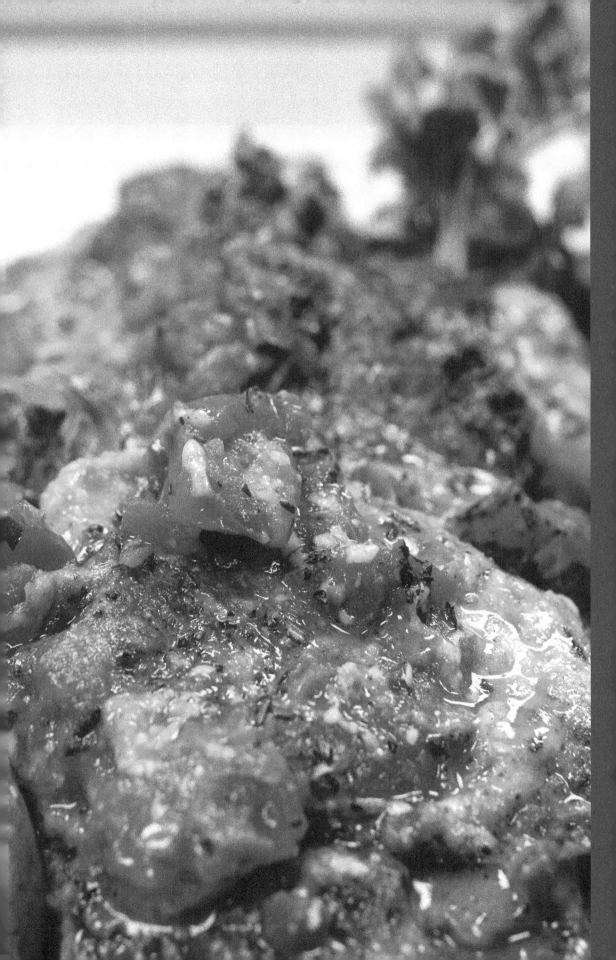

THE ULTIMATE LAMB SLIDER

Serves: 4

INGREDIENTS

2 Pounds of ground lamb

2 Teaspoons of minced garlic

5 Mint leaves *(rough chopped)*

1 Teaspoon of coriander

1 Teaspoon of seasoned salt

½ Teaspoon of ground curry powder

¼ Cup of Worcestershire sauce

12 Slider buns

DIRECTIONS

In a large bowl, combine the lamb and seasonings. Mix well and place in the refrigerator for about an hour. Using a small ice cream scoop, portion the sliders and form into a patty. The sliders can be grilled, baked in the oven at 375 for about 12 minutes or cooked in a skillet 3 minutes on each side until desired temperature is reached. Lamb shouldn't be cooked well done. Medium is the perfect temperature and slightly pink on the inside. Enjoy with your favorite condiments of mustard, steak sauce, ketchup, or mint jelly. The buns can be toasted as well.

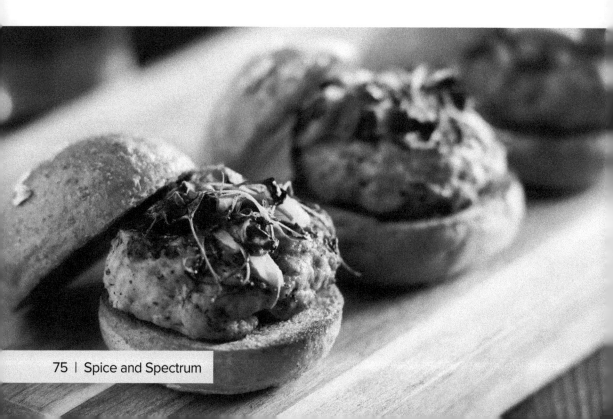

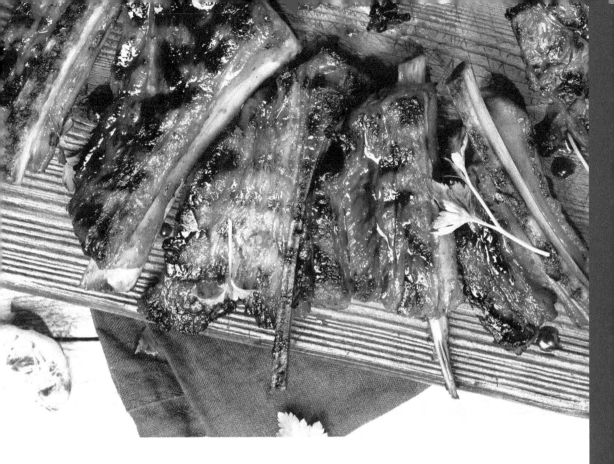

BBQ BEEF RIB

Serves: 4

INGREDIENTS

2 Slabs of beef ribs

1 Tablespoon of seasoned salt

2 Tablespoons of garlic powder

1 Tablespoons of smoked paprika

½ Tablespoon of ground black pepper

¼ Cup of vegetable oil

¼ Cup of water

¼ Cup of Worcestershire sauce

DIRECTIONS

Pre-heat the oven to 250. In a small bowl, combine the seasonings and mix well. Rub the oil over the ribs. Use the seasoning rub and season the ribs liberally. Place the ribs in a casserole dish. Add the water and Worcestershire sauce to the pan. Cover with foil and bake for 2 ½ hours or until tender. Enjoy!

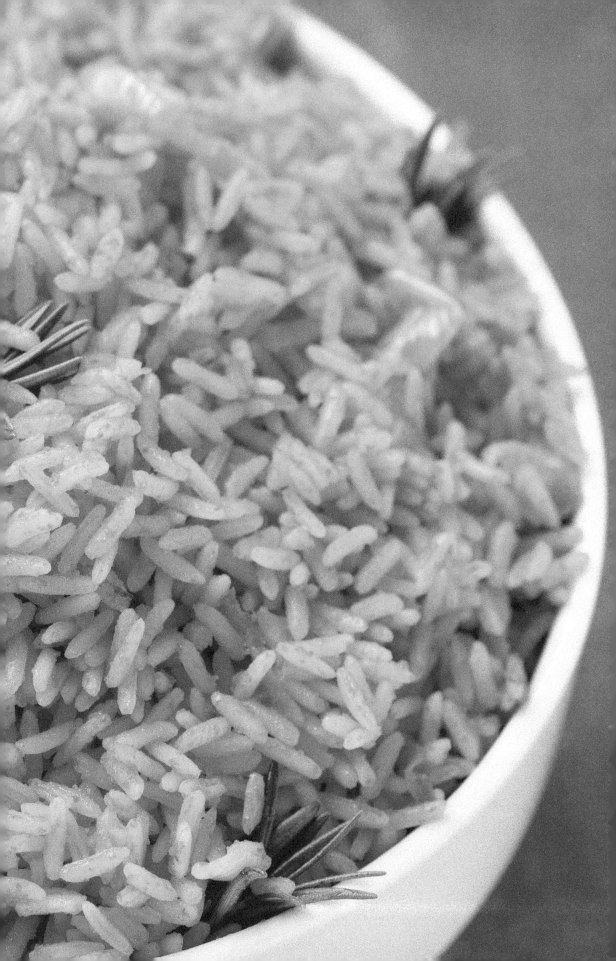

JOLLOF RICE

Serves: 4

INGREDIENTS

½ Cup of vegetable oil

2 Large red bell peppers *(diced)*

1 Large white onion

8 Garlic cloves *(chopped)*

5 Roma *(plum)* tomatoes *(large diced)*

½ Scotch bonnet pepper

2 Teaspoons of cayenne pepper

1 Teaspoon of dry thyme

2 Teaspoons of curry powder

1 Teaspoon of smoked paprika

2 Tablespoons of sugar

¼ Cup of hot sauce

1 Tablespoon of tomato paste

3 Cups of long grain rice

3 Cups of chicken or vegetable broth

DIRECTIONS

Place a large pot onto the stove on medium high. Add the oil to the pot. Once the oil is hot, add the bell peppers, onions, and garlic. Sauté for about 4 minutes. Add the tomatoes, scotch bonnet, cayenne, thyme, curry, and paprika. Stir well to prevent sticking. Cook for about 2 minutes. Add the remaining ingredients and mix well. Bring the pot to a boil. Cover with a lid and reduce the heat to low. Allow the rice to cook for about 20 minutes. Every so often, give the rice a good stir. Once the rice is cooked, remove the cover and flake with a fork. Serve as a side or add your favorite meat or seafood.

NOTE: 2 Pounds of meat *(chicken, beef, or shrimp)* can be added to the rice. The chicken or beef would be added with the tomatoes. The shrimp would be added during the last five minutes of cooking.

 The Motherland in a pan.

SOUTHERN BAKED CHICKEN

Serves: 8

INGREDIENTS

2 Whole chickens cut into 8 pieces each *(rinsed under cold water, drained well)*

1 Cup of olive oil

3 Tablespoons of rotisserie seasoning

1 Tablespoon of garlic powder

1 Tablespoon of black pepper

1 Tablespoon of seasoned salt

2 Teaspoons of dry thyme

2 Teaspoons of fresh chopped rosemary

1 Tablespoon of fresh chopped parsley

1 Tablespoon of ground coriander

½ Cup of all-purpose flour

½ Cup of vegetable oil

1 Small yellow onion *(chopped)*

3 Cups of chicken broth

DIRECTIONS

Pre-heat the oven to 350. In a large bowl, combine the oil, rotisserie seasoning, garlic, season salt, pepper, thyme, rosemary, parsley, and coriander. Mix well. Place the chicken in the seasoning mix. Be sure that all the chicken is covered liberally with the seasoning marinade. Cover with plastic wrap.

NOTE: This step can be done a day ahead of time. The longer the chicken marinades, the better the taste.

Remove the chicken from the marinade and place in a roasting pan. Pour any leftover marinade on top of the chicken. Cover with foil and a tight-fitting lid. Bake for about an hour and a half.

After the chicken comes out of the oven, place a large skillet onto the stove on medium high. Add the oil to the skillet and let it heat up. Once the oil is hot, whisk the flour into the oil. Continue whisking until it becomes lite brown. Remove the cover and foil from the chicken. Pour the broth of the chicken into the skillet. Continue stirring until no lumps remain. Once the gravy is smooth, pour the gravy over the chicken. Serve over rice or mashed potatoes.

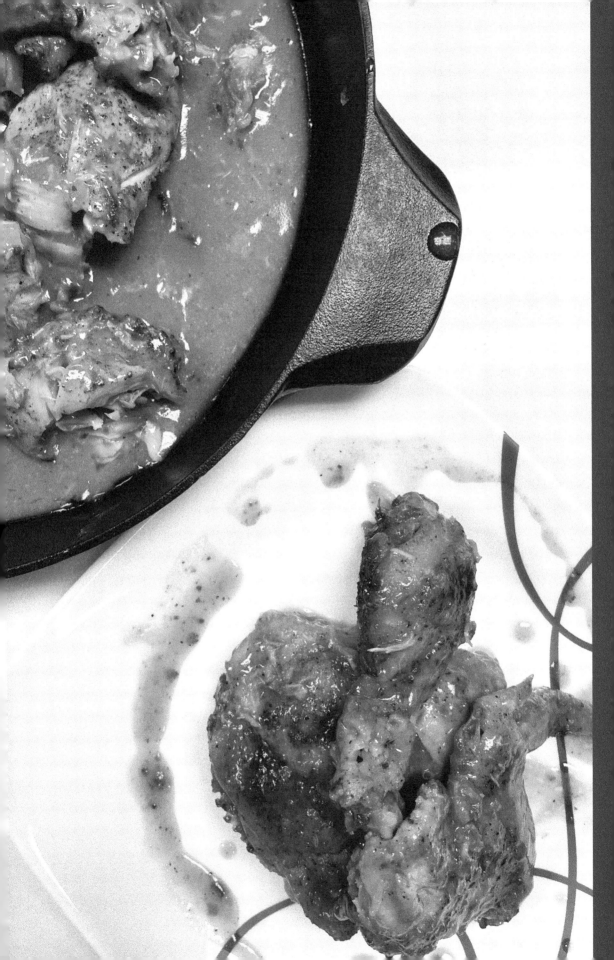

BBQ SHORT RIBS

Serves: 4

INGREDIENTS

BBQ SHORT RIBS

2 Cups of vegetable oil

½ Cup of all-purpose flour

2 Teaspoons of black pepper

3 Teaspoons of salt

2 Teaspoons of granulated garlic powder

2 Pounds of beef short ribs
(boneless or bone in)

1 Teaspoon of dry thyme flakes

1 Yellow onion (sliced)

2 Cups of beef broth

¼ Cup of Worcestershire sauce

BBQ SAUCE

2 Cups of ketchup

¼ Cup of sugar

¼ Cup of soy sauce

DIRECTIONS

Pre-heat the oven to 350. Place a large skillet onto the stove on medium high. Add the oil to the skillet and allow it to heat up for about 5 minutes.

In a medium size bowl, combine the flour, pepper, salt, and garlic powder. Mix well. Add the ribs to the flour and coat well. Place the ribs into the oil and brown on both sides. Cook for about 3 minutes on each side. Drain well.

Place the ribs into a large enough casserole dish. Add the thyme, onions, broth and Worcestershire sauce. Cover with foil and place the dish into the oven and cook for about 2 ½ hours. Remove the dish from the oven. The ribs should be fork tender and separated from the bone. In a small sauce pot, combine the ingredients for the bbq sauce and mix well. Place on the stove on medium high. Allow the sauce to come to a simmer. Stir occasionally to prevent sticking. Once the sugar is dissolved, remove from the heat and pour over the ribs. Return the ribs to the oven for 5 minutes. Place the ribs onto a platter or plate. Serve and enjoy!

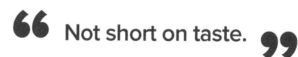 **Not short on taste.**

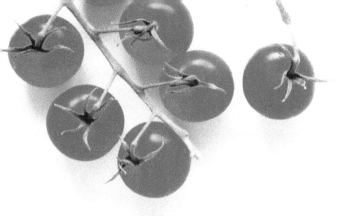
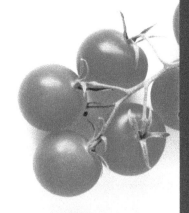

LINGUINI WITH TOMATO & BASIL SAUCE

Serves: 4

INGREDIENTS

1 Tablespoon of salt

½ Box of linguini noodles

2 Tablespoons of Olive oil

2 Tablespoons of sliced unsalted butter

1 Can of fire roasted tomatoes

½ Cup of half and half

2 Tablespoons of grated or fresh parmesan cheese

½ Cup of fresh basil leaves *(chopped)*

DIRECTIONS

Fill a large pot halfway with water. Place the pot onto the stove on high. Allow the water to come to a boil. Add the salt to the water. Immediately add the pasta to the boiling water. Using a pasta spoon or tongs, mix the pasta well for about 1 minute to prevent sticking. Allow the pasta to cook for about 7-8 minutes until done. Once the pasta has reached the desired tenderness, pour the pasta into a strainer and rinse under cold water. Drain well for about 5 minutes. Set aside for later use.

Place a large skillet onto the stove on medium high. Add the olive oil, butter and tomatoes. Sautee' for about 5 minutes. Add the half and half and continue to cook for a additional 3 minutes. Add the pasta to the skillet and toss well. Top with parmesan cheese and basil.

Note: This recipe can be served with your favorite chicken or seafood or can be eaten alone. Enjoy!

SKILLET BAKED CHICKEN & SALSA

Serves: 4

INGREDIENTS

½ Cup of all-purpose flour

1 Teaspoon of black pepper

½ Teaspoon of salt

1 Teaspoon of granulated garlic powder

1 Teaspoon of cumin

2 Tablespoons of olive oil

4 Large boneless, skinless, chicken breast cutlets *(rinsed under cold water and patted dry)*

1 Cup of your favorite salsa

½ Cup of Monterey Jack cheese

DIRECTIONS

Pre-heat the oven on 375. In a large mixing bowl, combine the flour with the salt, pepper, garlic, and cumin. Mix well. Place a large oven safe skillet onto the stove on medium high. Add the olive oil. Place the chicken into the flour mixture. Shake off the extra flour from the chicken and place the chicken into the skillet. Cook on both sides for about 4 minutes. Pour the salsa over the chicken and cover with foil. Place the chicken into the oven. Cook for about 15 minutes. Remove the skillet from the oven and remove the foil. Add the cheese over the chicken and return the skillet back to the oven. Melt the cheese for about 5 minutes. Enjoy!

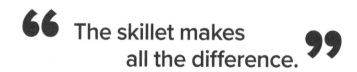

" The skillet makes all the difference. "

STOVE TOP STEAK

Serves: 4

INGREDIENTS

¼ Cup of olive oil

¼ Cup of Worcestershire sauce

1 Tablespoon of minced garlic

1 Tablespoon of onion powder

1 Teaspoon of black pepper

½ Cup of warm water

4 Ribeye steaks

DIRECTIONS

Use a small mixing bowl to combine all the ingredients. Mix well. Pour the mixture into a gallon size Ziploc bag. Add the steaks to the bag. Allow the steaks to marinade for at least an hour but no more than three days. Place a large skillet onto the stove on medium high. Try using a skillet that has a lid to cover. Remove the steaks from the bag and place into the skillet. Reserve the marinade. Do not overcrowd the pan. Cover the steaks with the lid or use aluminum foil.

Place a small pot on the stove on high heat. Pour the remaining marinade into the pot and bring to a boil. Once the sauce comes to a boil, reduce the heat to medium low. Allow the sauce to simmer for at least 20 minutes.

Allow the steaks to cook for about 4 minutes. Keep the steak covered while cooking. Turn the steak over and continue to cook for an additional 4 minutes. Once the steak has reached the desired temperature, remove the steaks from the skillet and place onto a platter. Let the steaks rest for about 5 minutes before cutting. Spoon the marinade over the steaks and enjoy.

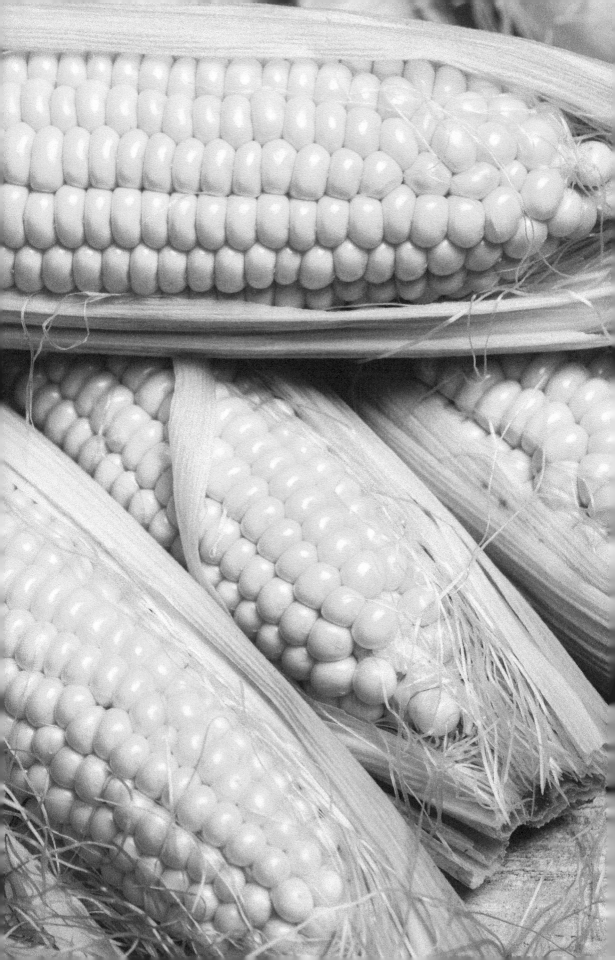

ROASTED CAJUN CORN

Serves: 6 – 8

INGREDIENTS

6 Ears of corn

1 Pound of butter

1 Tablespoon of garlic

1 Tablespoon of onion powder

¼ Cup of Worcestershire sauce

1 Tablespoon of Cajon seasoning

1 ½ Tablespoon of lite
brown sugar

¼ Cup of Tabasco sauce

¼ Cup of lemon juice

1 Tablespoon of chopped parsley
(fresh is best)

DIRECTIONS

Preheat your grill or oven to 350. Wash the corn and place into a casserole dish. Place a small sauce pot onto the stove on medium high. Add the ingredients into the pot and mix well. Bring the sauce to a simmer. Cook for about 10 minutes on low heat.

Use a pastry brush to coat the corn with the sauce. Place the corn into the oven. Cook for about 10 minutes. Rotate the corn and continue cooking for an additional 10 minutes. Remove the corn from the oven and add more sauce if you desire.

Place the corn on a platter and enjoy!

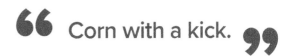 Corn with a kick.

SMOTHERED LIVER & SPINACH

Serves: 6

INGREDIENTS

1 Cup of vegetable oil

2 Pounds of calf liver
(cut into strips about an index finger length and width)

1 Cup of all-purpose flour

1 Teaspoon of salt

1 Teaspoon of pepper

1 Teaspoon of garlic powder

1 Yellow onion *(thin sliced)*

2 Tablespoons of salted butter

½ Tablespoon of lite brown sugar

¼ Cup of Worcestershire sauce

1 ¼ Cup of beef broth

½ Pound of spinach

DIRECTIONS

Place a large skillet on the stove on medium high. Pour the oil into the skillet to heat up. Cut the liver into strips. Combine the flour with the salt, pepper, and garlic. Mix well.

Place the liver into the flour and coat the liver well. Shake off the excess flour and put the liver into the skillet. Allow the liver to cook for about 4 minutes. Toss while cooking. Do not overcook the liver.

Remove the liver from the skillet and set aside. Place the onion into the skillet with the butter. Sautee for about 4 minutes. Add the brown sugar and mix until well blended. Add the liver back to the skillet with the Worcestershire sauce, the broth and the spinach. Fold the spinach into the mixture. Once the spinach is wilted, Add it over a bed of rice or mashed potatoes and enjoy!

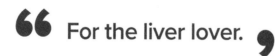 **For the liver lover.**

BAKED CHICKEN & RICE CASSEROLE

Serves: 4

INGREDIENTS

1 Whole chicken *(cut into 8 pieces)*

1 Cup of olive oil

2 Tablespoon of rotisserie seasoning

1 Teaspoon of salt

1 Teaspoon of black pepper

1 Teaspoon of garlic powder

1 Teaspoon of dry thyme

1 ½ Cup of rice

3 Cups of chicken broth

1 Can of Campbell's golden mushroom soup

1 Can of water *(from the soup can)*

1 Tablespoon of fresh chopped parsley

DIRECTIONS

Pre-heat the oven to 375. Wash the cut chicken pieces and drain well. Use paper towels to pat dry. In a large bowl, combine the oil, salt, pepper, garlic, and thyme. Mix well. Place the chicken pieces into the mix. Massage the seasonings into the chicken. Place the chicken into the refrigerator and marinade for at least one hour. Note: The longer the chicken marinade the better. 24 hours prior would be phenomenal.

Place the chicken in a large casserole dish. Cover the chicken with foil and bake for 45 minutes. Remove the chicken from the oven. Remove the chicken from the dish and set aside. Add the rice into the dish and spread evenly. Place the chicken back on top of the rice. Carefully pour the chicken broth over the rice and chicken. Cover with foil and continue to cook for an additional 40 minutes. In the meantime, combine the soup and water together. Cook the soup until its hot. Remove the dish from the oven. Pour the soup over the chicken. Return the dish to the oven and cook for 10 minutes. Sprinkle with parsley and serve. Enjoy!

 Not your mom's casserole.

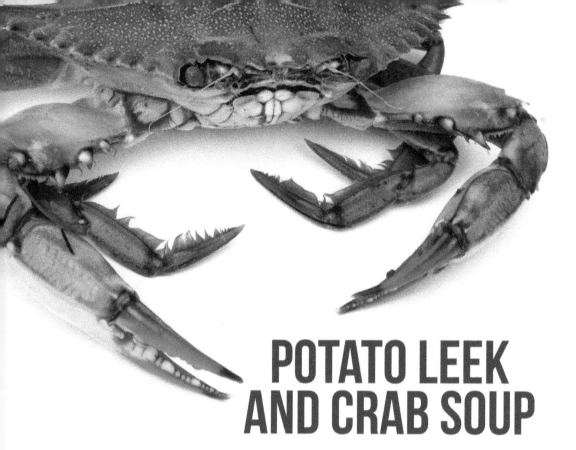

POTATO LEEK AND CRAB SOUP

Serves: 4

INGREDIENTS

1 Pound of white potatoes
(cut into bite size pieces)

4 Cups of chicken broth

2 Teaspoons of salt

1 Cup of heavy cream

1 ½ Tablespoons of vegetable oil

¼ Cup of chopped leeks

1 Tablespoon of minced garlic

1 Teaspoon of dry thyme

1 Teaspoon of white pepper

8oz Lump crab

DIRECTIONS

Place a large pot on the stove on medium high. Add the potatoes, broth, salt, and cream to the pot. Bring the potatoes to a boil. Reduce the heat to medium low.

Place a large skillet onto the stove on medium high. Add the oil, leeks, thyme, and pepper. Sauté for about 4 minutes. Add the vegetables to the pot of potatoes. Continue to cook until the potatoes are fork tender. Add the crab to the pot. Continue cooking for 10 minutes. Serve with garlic bread!

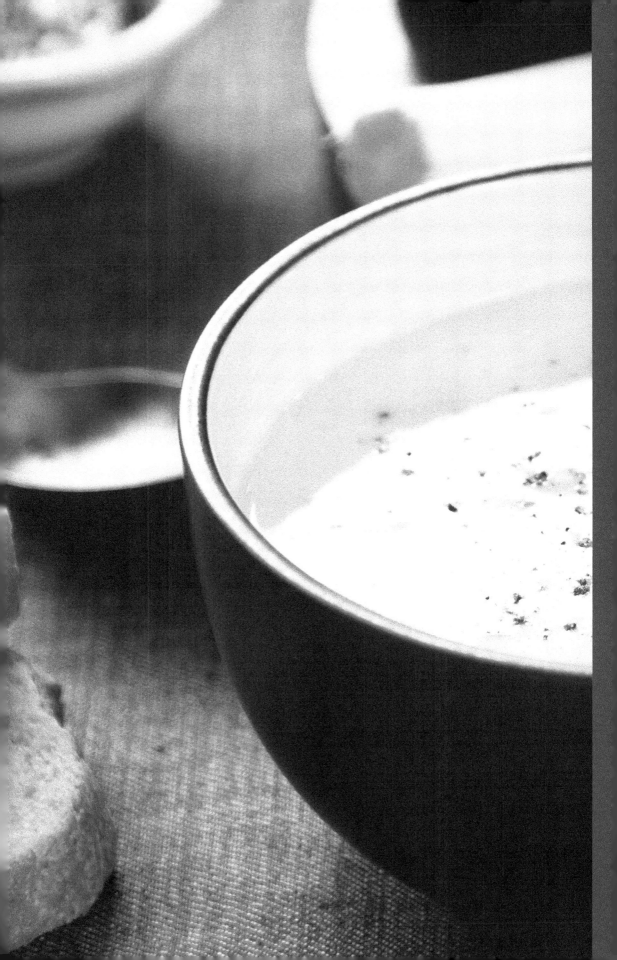

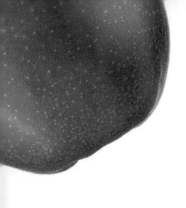
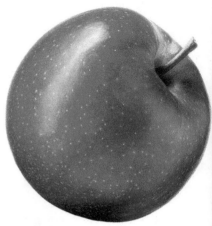

APPLE GLAZED
PORK TENDERLOIN

Serves: 4

INGREDIENTS

2 Pork tenderloins

2 Tablespoons of Dijon mustard

1 Teaspoon of salt

1 Teaspoon of pepper

1 Cup of purpose flour

¼ Cup of olive oil

2 Tablespoons of unsalted butter

1 Small red apple
(peeled and diced)

½ Cup of apple juice

DIRECTIONS

Pre-heat the oven to 350. Place a large oven proof skillet on the stove on medium high. Rinse the tenderloins under cold water. Use a small but sharp knife to remove any silver skin. Rub the mustard over the tenderloins. In a bowl, combine the salt, pepper, and flour. Mix well.

Add the oil and butter to the skillet. Coat the pork in the flour. Brown on all sides. Cook for about 4 minutes. Add the apples and the juice to the skillet. Place the skillet in the oven and cook for about 10 minutes. Remove the skillet from the oven. Let the pork rest for about 5 minutes before slicing. Serve over pasta, rice or potatoes.

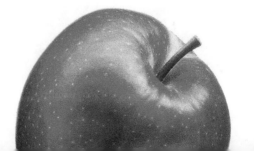

SWEET THAI SNAPPER

Serves: 4

INGREDIENTS

FRIED SNAPPER

2 Cups of vegetable oil

¼ Cup of sesame oil

4 Fresh red snapper filets

¾ Cup of all-purpose flour

1 Teaspoon of black pepper

2 Teaspoons of salt

SWEET THAI SAUCE

1 ½ Cup of rice wine vinegar

¼ Cup of lite soy sauce

3 Tablespoons of lite brown sugar

1 Small yellow onion *(thinly sliced)*

1 Tablespoon of minced garlic

1Teaspoon of crushed red pepper flakes

1 Tablespoon of fresh cilantro *(chopped)*

DIRECTIONS

FRIED SNAPPER

Pre-heat the oven to 425. Place a large skillet on the stove on medium high. Add the oils to the skillet. Score the snapper (cut slits) two or three times. In a mixing bowl, combine the flour, salt, and pepper. Place the snapper into the oil. Cook on both sides for about 4 minutes each. Remove the snapper from the pan and place into a casserole dish. Set aside for later use.

SWEET THAI SAUCE

In a small mixing bowl, combine all the ingredients. Mix well. Pour the sauce over the fish and place the casserole dish into the oven. Bake the fish for about 10 minutes. Remove the fish from the oven and place on a platter. Serve with coconut rice. Garnish with fresh cilantro.

 Oh snap, that's sweet!

OXTAIL RAGU OVER PAPPARDELLE PASTA

Serves: 4

INGREDIENTS

½ Cup of olive oil

2 Teaspoons of salt

2 Teaspoons of black pepper

1 Cup of all-purpose flour

3 Pounds of beef oxtails

1 Large yellow or white onion

1 Tablespoon of minced garlic

¼ Cup of Worcestershire sauce

3 Cups of tomato sauce

3 Cups of beef broth or enough to cover the oxtails

5 Fresh sprigs of thyme

2 Sprigs of fresh rosemary

DIRECTIONS

Place a 5-quart pot onto the stove on medium high. In a large bowl, combine the salt, pepper, and flour. Add the oil to the pot. Coat the oxtails in the flour and place them in the pot.

Brown the oxtails on all sides. Cook for about 7 minutes. Add the remaining ingredients and bring to a boil. Once the pot comes to a boil, cover with a tight-fitting lid. Reduce the heat to low. Simmer the oxtails for about 3 hour or until the oxtails are fork tender.

While the oxtails are cooking, fill a medium size pot with water and place it onto the stove. Bring to a boil and cook the pasta according to the directions on the box.

Once the pasta is finished cooking, drain the pasta and rinse with cold water. Add a little oil to prevent from sticking.

As the oxtails finish cooking, remove the pot and place it on a cooler part of the stove. Let sit for about an hour. Skim off the excess fat from the oxtails. If possible, prepare this dish a day before serving. It'll make the fat easier to remove when cold.

Once you're ready to reheat the oxtails, slowly bring the oxtails back up to temperature. Place a large skillet onto the stove. Add the sauce to the skillet. Add pasta to the sauce and sauté until the pasta and sauce is hot. Serve immediately!

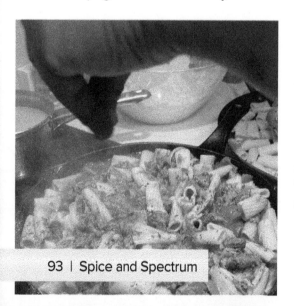

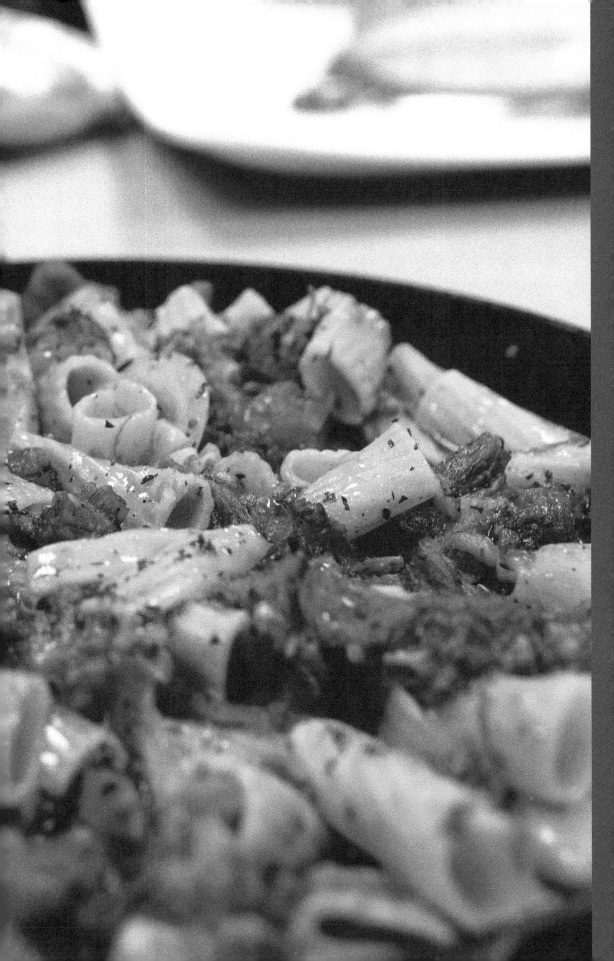

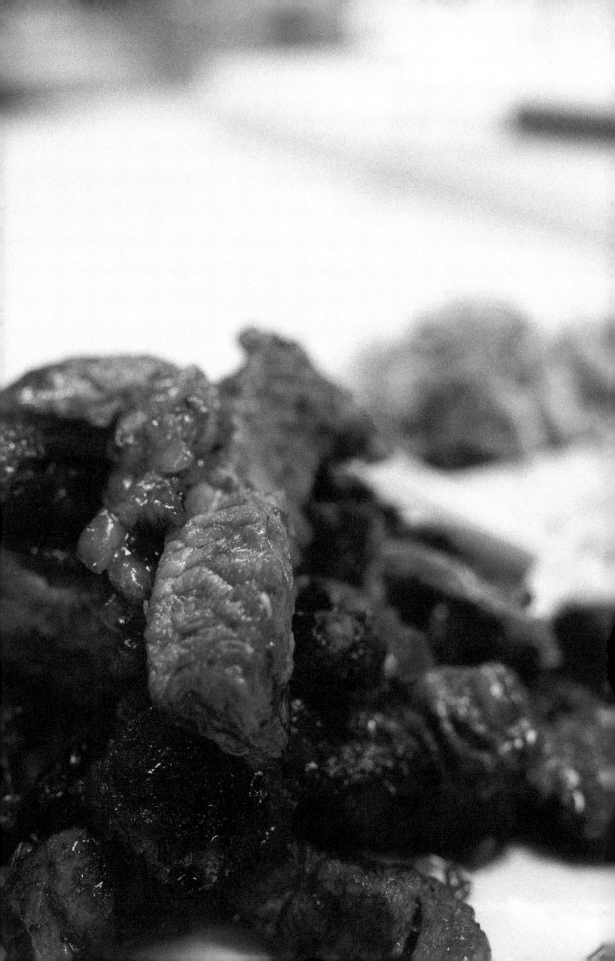

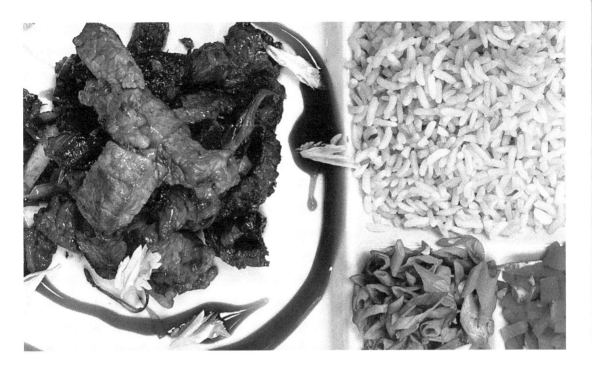

KOREAN BEEF
& BROWN RICE

Serves: 4

INGREDIENTS

4 Ribeye steaks *(very thinly sliced)*

¾ Cups of soy sauce

1 Tablespoon of minced garlic

1 Tablespoon of chopped ginger

2 Tablespoons of lite brown sugar

1 ½ Teaspoons of red pepper flakes

1 Small yellow onion *(thinly sliced)*

3 Stalks of scallions *(chopped)*

2 Tablespoons of toasted sesame oil

2 Cups of brown rice

DIRECTIONS

In a bowl or casserole dish, combine the soy sauce, garlic, ginger, sugar, pepper flakes, onions, and sesame oil. Mix well. Add the steak to the mixture and rub throughout the meat. Marinade the steak for at least 4 hours. Overnight will yield the best success.

Prepare the rice according to the directions on the package. Place a large skillet onto the stove on high. Once the skillet is hot, add the steak to the pan. Cook for about 5 minutes. Stir well while the steak is in the pan. Serve the steak over the rice. Enjoy!

SAVORY BEEF & NOODLES

Serves: 8

INGREDIENTS

1 Pound of egg noodles

½ Tablespoon of olive oil

2 Pounds of beef tenderloin steak *(cut into bite size pieces)*

1 Whole yellow onion *(thin sliced)*

1 Tablespoon on minced garlic

Pinch of crushed red pepper flakes

1 Tablespoon of Cajon seasoning

1 Tablespoon of brown sugar

¼ Cup of Worcestershire sauce

½ Stick of butter *(unsalted) (melted)*

2 Tablespoons of fresh chopped parsley

DIRECTIONS

Prepare the noodles according to the directions on the package. Add the olive oil and toss well. Set aside until later use. Place a large skillet onto the stove on medium high. Add the steak, onion, pepper flakes, and Cajon seasoning. Sauté for about 2 ½ minutes. Add the brown sugar, Worcestershire sauce, and butter. Continue to cook for about 2 minutes. Add a serving of pasta to the center of the plate. Spoon a heaping serving of the steak in the center of the pasta. Garnish with the fresh parsley and enjoy!

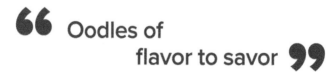

66 Oodles of flavor to savor 99

PISTACHIO CRUSTED LAMB CHOP FINISHED WITH A WILD BLUEBERRY SAUCE

Serves: 4

INGREDIENTS

LAMB CHOPS

2 Racks of lamb chops

2 ½ Tablespoons of Dijon mustard

1 Cup of chopped pistachios *(grind in a food processer until fine crumbs)*

1 Tablespoon of fresh chopped rosemary

1 Tablespoon of fresh chopped thyme

1 Tablespoon of minced garlic

1 Tablespoon of ground coriander

½ Tablespoon of cracked black pepper

2 Tablespoons of olive oil

WILD BLUEBERRY SAUCE

1 Cup of olive oil

½ Pint of fresh blueberries

½ Tablespoon of brown sugar

2 Tablespoons of melted butter

¼ Cup of Worcestershire sauce

DIRECTIONS

Pre-heat the oven to 425 or grill to 375. Rinse the lamb of under cold water to rid the excess blood. Pat dry with a paper towel. Apply the mustard over the top part of the lamb liberally. Season the lamb with the pistachios, rosemary, thyme, garlic, coriander, and black pepper. This will create a crust.

Drizzle the olive oil over the crust. Wrap the lamb in plastic and place in the refrigerator for about an hour. In the meantime, prepare the sauce.

Place a sauce pot onto the stove on medium high. Combine the oil and blueberries. Simmer for about 5 minutes until the berries began to burst. Add the brown sugar. Stir and continue to cook. Stir in the butter and Worcestershire sauce. Continue to simmer for about 5 minutes. Set aside for later use. Remove the lamb from the refrigerator and remove the plastic wrap. Place the lamb onto a sheet pan or casserole dish and place in the oven or on the grill. Cook for about 10 minutes or until desired temperature is reached...

Remove the lamb from the oven or grill. Allow the lamb to rest before slicing. Drizzle the sauce over the lamb and serve with your favorite side.

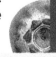

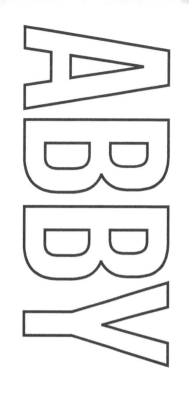

It is the soul of West Africa, the warm, spicy tapestry of flavors, the heart of Abby's mom, that make the dishes uniquely their own.

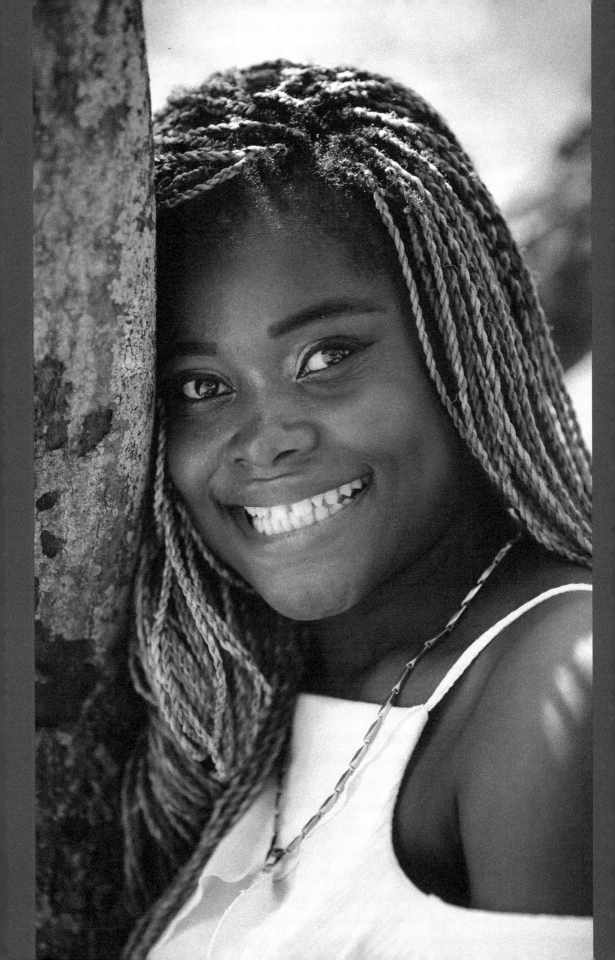

ABBY

Abby, whose name is Americanized from an African name, Folayemi, is a senior at iCan Dream Center. Abby comes from a West African family and Jamaican heritage. A native of Benin, Abby's mother prepares traditional African meals for the family. Fufu (pounded yam), curry goat soup, Jollof rice, Bissap tea, and addictive Mandazis (African donuts) are just some of the foods that Abby enjoys with Mr. Matt, who is a connoisseur of her family's cuisine.

Matt commonly asks Abby, "What were you having for dinner last night?" She describes eating Egusi, a stew traditionally eaten by scooping it out of a bowl using fufu with her family gathered around. During the conversation, her classmates listen attentively. The style of cooking inherent in African cuisine is spice-driven and flavorful, but it also embodies simple culinary techniques that Abby has internalized. The students cook familiar dishes at iCan Dream, such as soups, stews, breads, bowls, hand-helds, and grilled meats since they are familiar with them.

Although Abby's dinner table is influenced by a heavy cultural influence, the menu is very different from what her classmates eat at home. She enjoys the delicacies of American teenage cuisine. Hot Cheetos, Oreos, and hot wings are among her favorites. However, for Abby, home-cooked food serves as a safe and irresistible catalyst for conversation. In this way, she can create a balance between her West African upbringing and her identity as a young American teenager. This encourages her to embrace her heritage as well as exalts it while at the same time providing her with the soft and familiar edges required to simply fit in.

Mr. Matt relates a discussion about curry goat back to a lesson about the Dahomey Warriors, an all-female regiment in Dahomey. Today, this country is known as Benin. That is where Abby's mother acquired her culinary skills. This is the same place where her grandmother learned to cook. Additionally, Abby enjoys the jerk flavors of Jamaican cuisine. An homage to her father's homeland, she has prepared business plans for opening and running her own restaurant in Jamaica. Over the years, she has watched quietly, tasting each layer as it was added to create the perfect balance of heat and sweetness, coconut milk, curry, jerk, etc.

You should watch out, Folayemi will not be modest about the spice in her name, she will demand that the legacy of her name be honored in whatever she does.

66 Although Abby's dinner table is influenced by a heavy cultural influence, the menu is very different from what her classmates eat at home. She enjoys the delicacies of American teenage cuisine. Hot Cheetos, Oreos, and hot wings are among her favorites. However, for Abby, home-cooked food serves as a safe and irresistible catalyst for conversation. In this way, she can create a balance between her West African upbringing and her identity as a young American teenager. 99

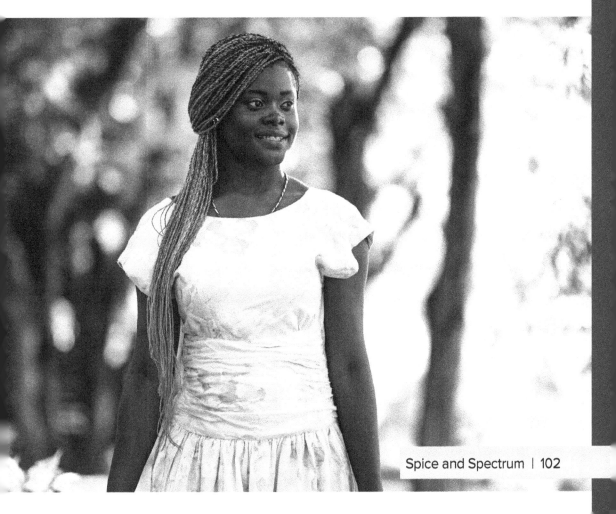

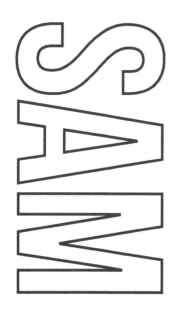

SAM

While there is plenty of dignity and honor in a job where janitorial services are performed, folks with learning disabilities are frequently marginalized into those opportunities.

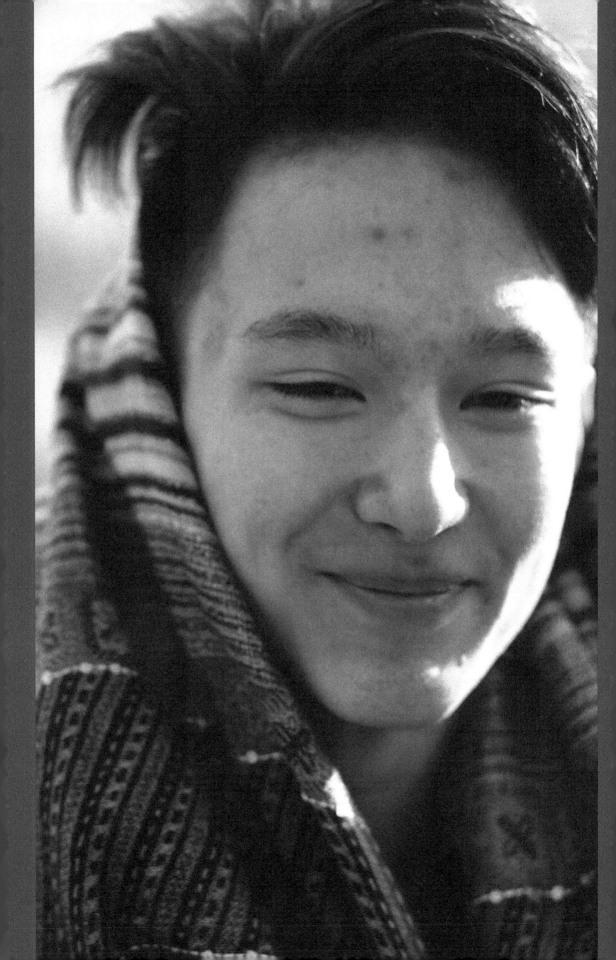

SAM

It is common for teens and young adults to have unhealthy eating habits. Through culinary classes, students can learn healthy recipe ideas and become interested in the cooking process. This in turn encourages teens to make healthier lifestyle choices.

When Sam first came to iCan Dream Center, he was a 17-year-old high school junior with an obsession with French fries and soft drinks. Sam is a 21-year-old student in our transition program for 18-22-year-olds who has completed many years of culinary courses.

The students were introduced to gourmet fare by Chef Jerome when he visited the center to introduce them to gourmet fare. Sam recalled that over the years, he had shifted from craving salty fried food to freshly prepared and flavorful dishes made by Miss Zipporah. Sam now appreciates how better food makes him feel, from salmon and rice to spaghetti and salad.

There is an emphasis on healthy, nutritious foods in culinary class, but that does not mean our students are unfamiliar with Ms. Z's famous peach cobbler or homemade caramel muffins. Sam has been able to apply that lesson to his life, as it is something many of the students need to learn. Sam has been able to live a healthier life by making smarter food choices and experimenting with new foods he might not have done otherwise. As well, he has expanded his social experience with food by trying out new dishes that he might not have otherwise tried.

Eating, however, is not the only aspect of the program. As students count, weigh, measure, and keep track of time, they practice various academic skills, including basic mathematics. Biology (where food originates from) and chemistry (how high temperatures can alter food items or how an egg yolk changes its structure while being whipped) are introduced. Cooking classes also allow students to gain social skills, as they work in teams and communicate in the kitchen. Students are exposed to a variety of kitchen technology and equipment.

Cooking classes are not just a tool to build the confidence of youth, they are designed for that purpose. Students feel a sense of accomplishment after completing a cooking class. The tangible results of the students' efforts enhance their sense of accomplishment. In addition, some of them can cook at home and are glad to assist their parents with the cooking routine, and even offer their own opinions. One thing we have found repeatedly is that cooking enhances work ethic.

As a result of their involvement in tasks in the kitchen related not only to cooking, but also to safety and cleanup procedures, students with disabilities develop a sense of responsibility. These students become more independent in their work practices. For instance, they can cook for themselves without asking someone for assistance. When a student like Sam unleashes his creative talents, it is one of the true joys in cooking class. Sam has, over the years, tested his creativity and experimented with the recipes contained within these pages.

Chef Rome taught Sam how to make a simple sauce or salad dressing, as well as how to make something decadent and special, such as suppertime casseroles. Sam has strengthened his palate, his imagination, and his self-care skills. The culinary class is also an impressively diverse experience for the students as they learn about other cultures from their peers as well as from guest chefs; all the while, they advance their studies by learning about international cuisines. As a result of this information, the students always develop an open-mindedness that takes them on an exciting journey of exploring new tastes, such as when Sam first tried couscous and learned that it was pasta.

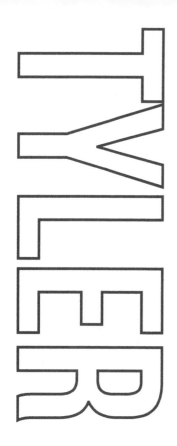

TYLER

Memories emanate from the food our families make and take on a life of their own.

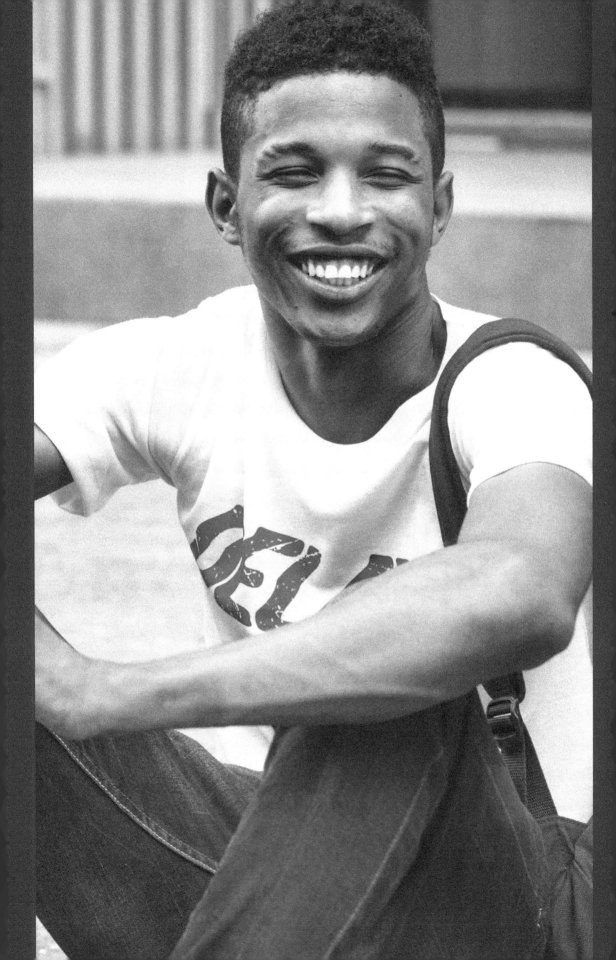

TYLER

Tyler is a post-secondary student who has come to iCan Dream. It is imperative that he learn how to develop essential academic and functional skills that will lead to meaningful community employment, and equally important, how to take care of himself daily. To put it simply, Tyler came to us to learn how to become an adult. He is doing a great job.

Tyler enjoys celebrating Christmas. The holiday brings him a sense of family and warmth. On Christmas day, his family always shares the same meal: jerk chicken, candied yams, cornbread, and lots of sweets. And just one smell of spaghetti instantly conjures a bittersweet feeling of both sorrow and fondness as Tyler's late father made the very best spaghetti. Tyler said, "When Ms. Zipporah taught me how to make spaghetti, I smiled because now I feel good when I cook spaghetti for my mom and sister, just like my dad made it for me.

Making a meal for someone is taking care of them. "That makes me feel happy to take care of someone I love."

Memories emanate from the food our families make and take on a life of their own. How amazing that these memories touch the senses of taste, touch, smell, and poignantly for Tyler, the sense of enduring love and happy familiarity in his heart.

66 Tyler's late father made the very best spaghetti... Memories emanate from the food our families make and take on a life of their own. How amazing that these memories touch the senses of taste, touch, smell, and poignantly for Tyler, the sense of enduring love and happy familiarity in his heart. **99**

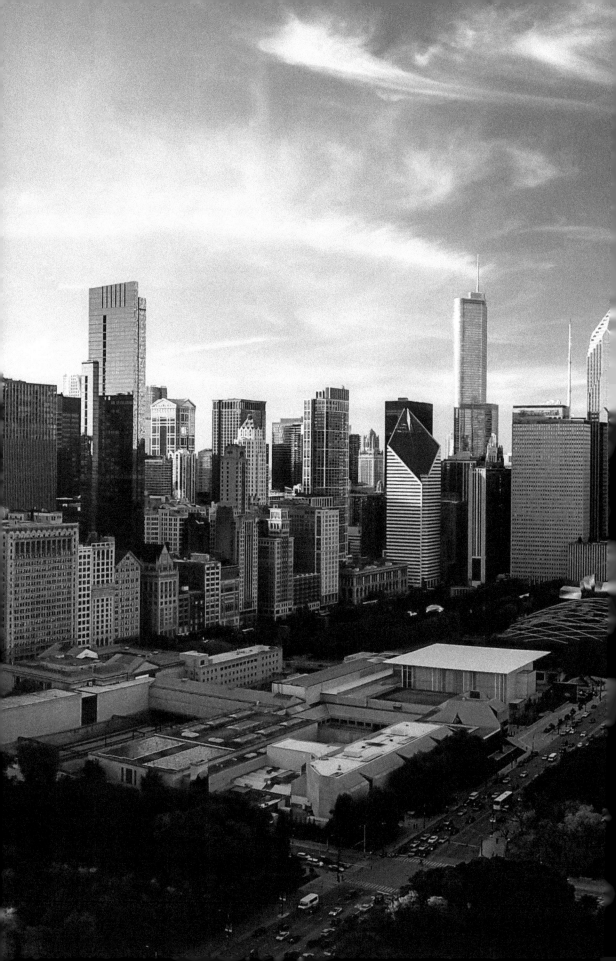

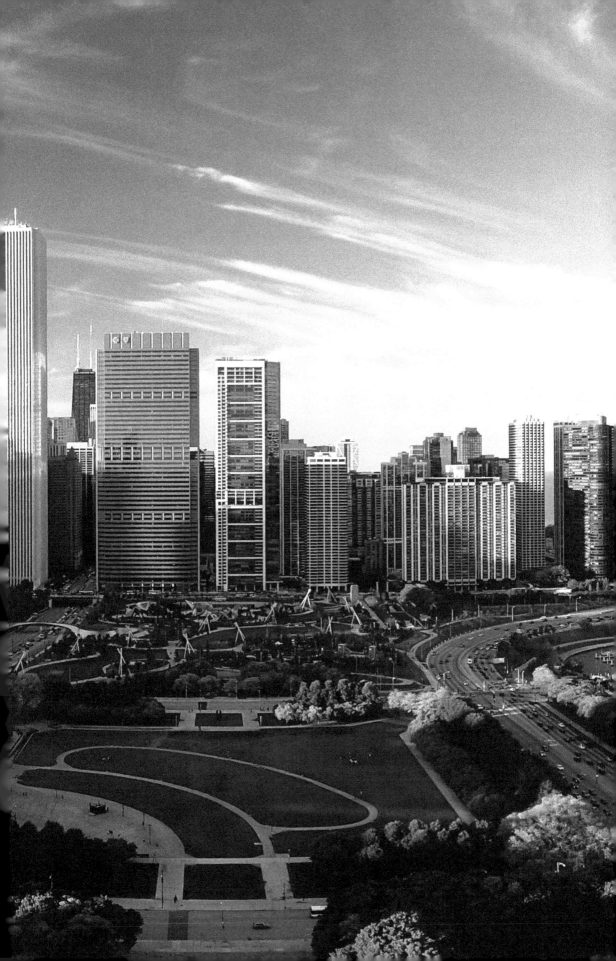

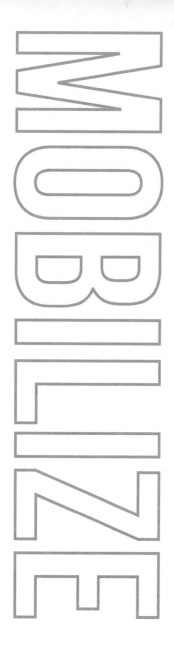

MOBILIZE

We encourage students to dream, but more significantly, we steer them towards realizing their dreams by guiding them through actionable steps.

Asian Honey and Salmon

A Simple Dip

Sauteed Shrimp Cakes

New Orleans Chicken Patties

Surf and Turf Stir Fry

Lemon Chicken Sauté

Lump Crab Sliders

Smokey Bacon Vinaigrette

Shrimp Risotto

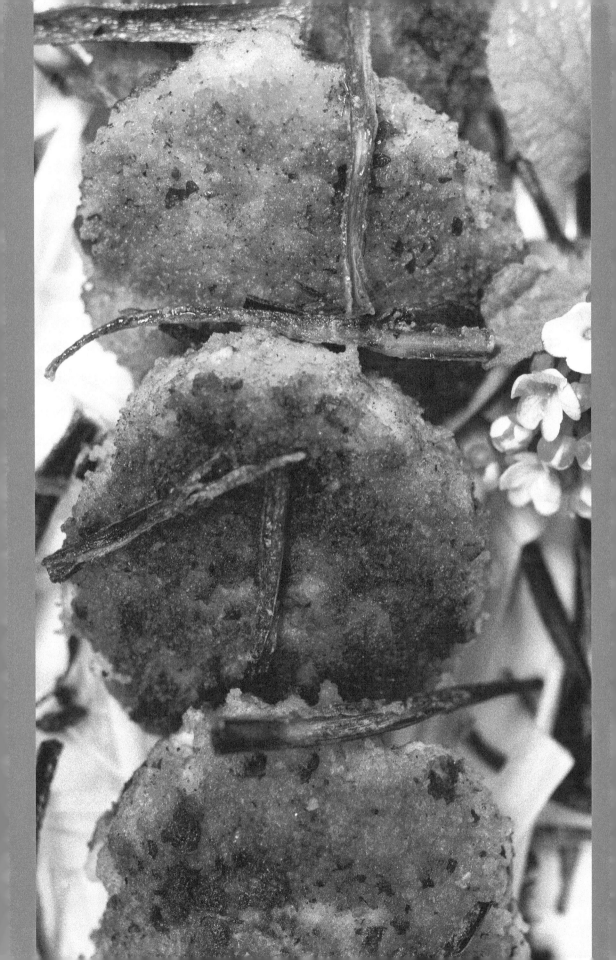

MOBILIZE

iCan Dream Center is a grassroots organization founded in March 2013 to fill a gap in disability services within South Cook and Will County, Illinois. We specialize in working with students with intellectual disabilities, autism, and various learning difficulties. The iCan Dream Center provides quality programming and a space for students to dream.

iCan Dream Center is a therapeutic school that is approved by the Illinois State Board of Education. We are unique in that we strive to provide an alternative-to-alternative schools. To date, alternative schools have mainly served as settings where more restrictive conditions are enforced to compensate for dangerous or disruptive behavior. There are inherent risks associated with not responding to the overwhelming reality that punitive settings are further crippling and (re)traumatizing our youth when we do not respond to the data.

What does the data say? Cumulatively, nearly 1 in 10 children entering 3rd grade experience placement in a disciplinary alternative school by 12th grade. What is the problem? There is a high risk in placing students in punitive alternative schools. There are systematically related predictors that are linked to the risk of subsequent juvenile detention. These predictors can be observed in early childhood and well into secondary school. We understand that alternative settings are often the "to" in the school to prison pipeline which is why we have taken an entirely different approach.

Trauma research suggests that as acceptance of the child grows, so does the progress of development in the child's areas of opportunity. The iCan Dream Center surrounds every student, regardless of their history, with a team of therapists, teachers and leaders who are on the same page and committed to maximizing the opportunities for growth. That page requires that we are unconditionally positive about the student's future and intentions with us. That page requires that our team accept the student's social-emotional journey as our own, thereby creating a community that is uplifting and always creating ways to innovate for the student.

The philosophical approach at iCan Dream Center is to foster growth in resiliency, skill building, self-discipline, maturity, mental health, and a growth mindset. The high expectations and loving supports empower students with challenging behaviors. There is massive value in making changes to the way we treat our youth.

iCan Dream Center has a unique niche in that we serve students who have mostly mild to moderate disabilities. Our students integrate into society without the need for braille, wheelchair access or a communication device. The fact that their intellectual processing, emotional, and social deficits are invisible creates a vulnerability, in the absence of interventions, to "typical" expectations in the workforce, when encountering law enforcement or in social situations. iCan Dream Center serves students with the capacity to maintain competitive employment. All our individualized planning and tailored support services are developed to **MOBILIZE** student success in the workforce (and life!) when they exit services.

We encourage students to dream, but more significantly, we steer them toward realizing their dreams by guiding them through actionable steps, not unlike the steps one takes following the recipes in this cookbook.

66 We understand that alternative settings are often the "to" in the school to prison pipeline which is why we have taken an entirely different approach. 99

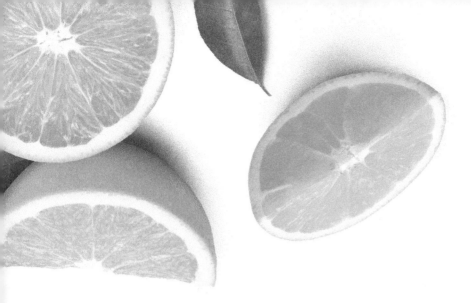

ASIAN HONEY
& ORANGE SALMON

Serves: 4

INGREDIENTS

4 Salmon filets

1 Teaspoon of salt

1 Teaspoon of cracked black pepper

2 Tablespoons of sesame oil

1 Jar of orange marmalade

Pinch of crushed red pepper flakes

1 Tablespoon of Dijon mustard

1 Tablespoon of lite soy sauce

1 Tablespoon of honey

Black sesame seed

1 Tablespoon of chopped scallions

DIRECTIONS

Place a large skillet on the stove on medium high. Allow the skillet to get hot. Season the salmon with salt and pepper. Add the oil to the skillet. Immediately place the skillet seasoned side down. Allow the salmon to cook for about 4 minutes. Turn the salmon over and continue to cook for another 3 minutes or so. Remove the salmon from the skillet and set on a plate or platter. Add to the skillet the marmalade, pepper flakes, mustard, soy sauce, honey and sesame seeds. Stir until mixed well. Spoon the sauce over the salmon. Garnish with the chopped scallions.

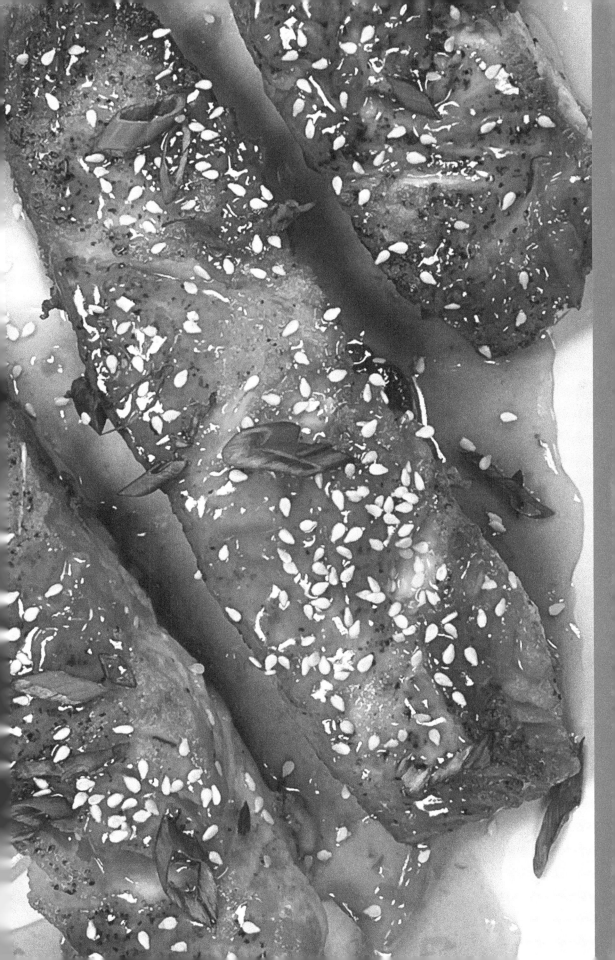

NEW ORLEANS CHICKEN PATTIES

Serves: 8 – 10

INGREDIENTS

2 Large boneless/skinless chicken breast *(small diced or chopped)*

1 Teaspoon of Cajun seasoning

1 Small yellow onion

2 Teaspoon of minced garlic

1 Small red and green bell pepper *(chopped)*

2 Teaspoons of Dijon mustard

1 Egg

1 Tablespoon of chopped parsley *(fresh)*

¼ Cup of plain breadcrumbs

½ Cup of olive oil

1 Stick of unsalted butter

DIRECTIONS

Rinse the chicken under cold water and pat dry with paper towel. Place the chicken in a bowl. Add the remaining ingredients except for the oil and butter. Mix well. Place the mixture into the refrigerator for about 10 minutes.

Place a large skillet onto the stove over medium high. Add the oil and butter to the skillet. Remove the mixture from the refrigerator and form into patties. Use an ice cream scoop for consistency. Carefully place the patties into the oil. Cook on each side for about 2 ½ minutes. Turn the patties over and repeat the step. Drain the patties on a paper towel. Serve immediately.

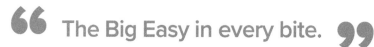 The Big Easy in every bite.

A SIMPLE DIP

Serves: 4

INGREDIENTS

2 Cans of whole kernel corn

1 Can of black beans

1 Can of fire roasted tomatoes

1 Small purple onion *(chopped)*

1 Chopped jalapeno
(chopped, seeds removed)

1 Tablespoon of chopped cilantro

½ Cup of house Italian dressing

DIRECTIONS

In a small bowl, combine all the ingredients and mix well. Cover and place into the refrigerator and chill until ready for use. Serve with your favorite tortilla.

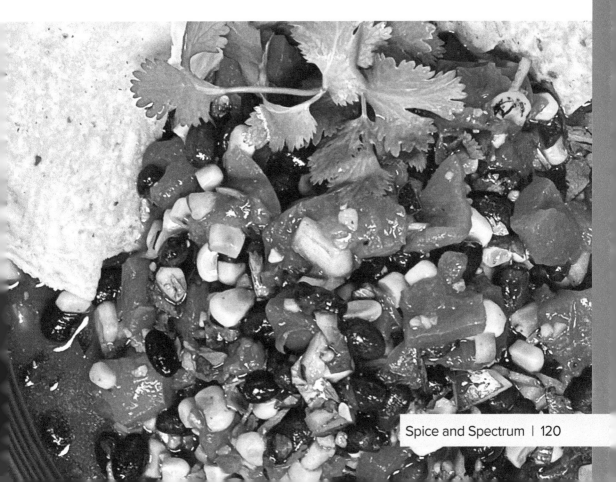

SAUTÉED SHRIMP CAKES

Serves: 4

INGREDIENTS

1 Cup of chopped shrimp

1 Teaspoon of Cajun seasoning

1 Teaspoon of garlic powder

1 Tablespoon of chopped
yellow onion

1 Tablespoon of lemon juice

½ Tablespoon of fresh
chopped parsley

½ Tablespoon of all-purpose flour

1 Egg

½ Cup of panko breadcrumbs

½ Cup of vegetable oil or olive oil

DIRECTIONS

In a large bowl, combine the shrimp, seasonings, flour, and egg. Mix well. Place the mixture into the refrigerator and chill for about 10 minutes. In the meantime, place the breadcrumbs into a small bowl or plate. Place a large skillet onto the stove over medium high. Remove the mixture from the refrigerator. Using a large ice-cream scoop, portion out the shrimp mixture and for into the shape of a patty. Coat each patty with the breadcrumbs and place into the skillet. Allow each shrimp cake to cook for about 3 ½ minutes on each side. Place the cakes on a paper towel lined plate to drain. Enjoy!

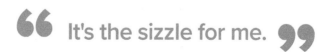

66 It's the sizzle for me. **99**

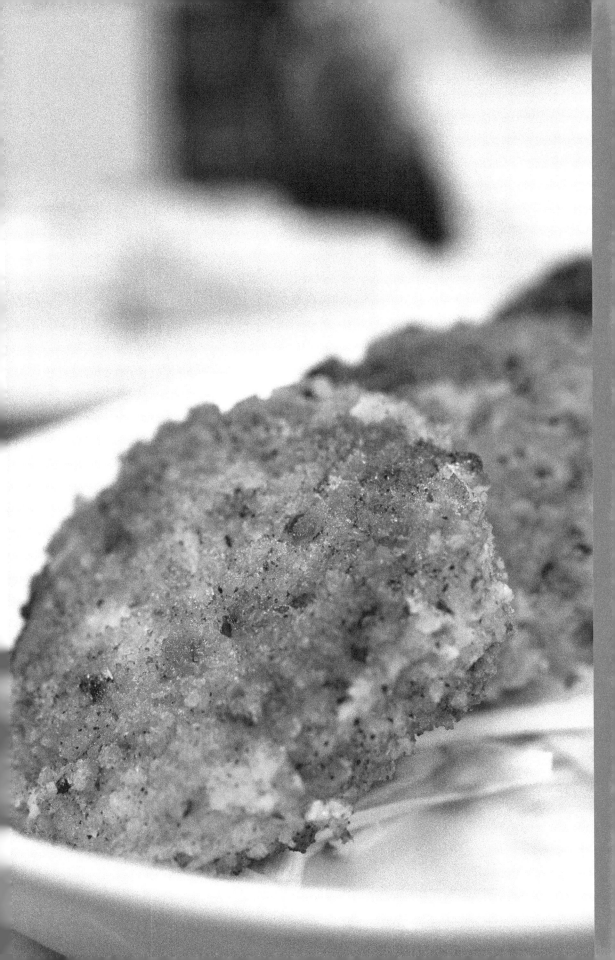

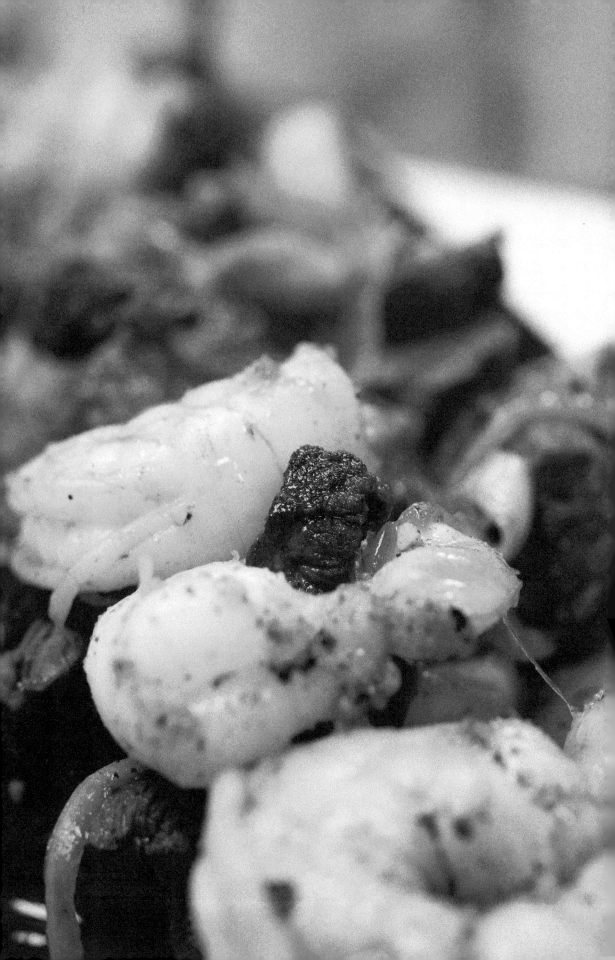

SURF & TURF STIR FRY

Serves: 4

INGREDIENTS

2 Thick ribeye steaks
(cut into strips)

2 Tablespoons of sesame oil

1 Red bell pepper *(cut into strips)*

1 Small onion *(cut into strips)*

10 Broccoli crowns

½ Pound of shrimp *(size 16/20, tail-off, peeled and deveined)*

1 Teaspoon of chopped ginger

1 Teaspoon of chopped garlic

1 Tablespoon of hoisin sauce

1 Tablespoon of oyster sauce

DIRECTIONS

Place a large skillet or wok onto the stove on medium high. Once the skillet has gotten hot, add the oil and steak. Cook the steak for about 3 minutes. Add the vegetables and continue cooking for an additional 3 minutes. Add the shrimp, ginger, garlic, and sauces. Cook for about 4 minutes. Do not overcook the shrimp. Serve over rice or eat it as is.

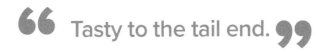 **" Tasty to the tail end. "**

LEMON CHICKEN SAUTÉ

Serves: 6

INGREDIENTS

½ Cup of all-purpose flour

1 Teaspoon of salt

1 Teaspoon of pepper

1 Teaspoon of granulated garlic powder

6 Boneless skinless chicken breasts

½ Cup of olive oil

Juice of one lemon

Zest of one lemon

1 Cup of chicken broth

1 Tablespoon of fresh chopped parsley

DIRECTIONS

Place a large skillet onto the stove on medium high. In a bowl, combine the flour, salt, pepper, and garlic. Mix well. Add the olive oil to the skillet. Coat the chicken in the flour mixture and carefully place the breasts into the skillet. Sauté' for 4 minutes on each side. Add the lemon juice, zest, and chicken broth. Continue cooking. After about 3 minutes, or until the sauce thickens. Once the sauce thickens, remove from the skillet. Serve over rice. Garnish with the parsley and enjoy!

LUMP CRAB SLIDERS

Serves: 8

INGREDIENTS

1 Pound of lump crab

½ Tablespoon of spicy brown mustard

1 Tablespoon of mayo

1 Tablespoon of lemon juice

1 Teaspoon of garlic powder

½ Tablespoon of Worcestershire sauce

A couple of dashes of tabasco sauce

1 Tablespoon of melted butter

2 Tablespoons of breadcrumbs

16 Slider rolls

1 Cup or hand full of bib lettuce

2 Teaspoons of olive oil

2 Teaspoons of white wine vinegar

DIRECTIONS

Use a fork to gently break up the crab meat. Combine all the ingredients in a bowl and mix well.

Place the mixture in the refrigerator for about 10 minutes. Place a skillet on the stove on medium high. Add about a ¼ cup of vegetable oil to the skillet. Use a 1 ½ ice cream scoop to portion out the crab cakes. Gently form and shape the cake. Place the crab cake into the pan and sear on both sides for about 2 ½ minutes. Once the crab cakes are finished cooking, place between the slider rolls. Mix the green and vinegar together and place on top the crab cakes.

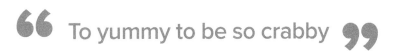
" To yummy to be so crabby "

SMOKEY BACON VINAIGRETTE

Serves: 4

INGREDIENTS

2 Slices of bacon *(cut into strips)*

1 Shallot *(chopped)*

½ Cup of champagne vinegar

2 Teaspoons of granulated garlic powder

1 Teaspoon of black pepper

3 Tablespoons of sugar

3 Tablespoons of your favorite dry rub

1 Tablespoon of Worcestershire sauce

DIRECTIONS

Place a large skillet onto the stove over medium high. Sauté the bacon and shallot. Cook the bacon until done. Place the bacon, shallots, and bacon grease into a blender. Add the remaining ingredients and blend for about 30 seconds. Allow the dressing to cool. Pour into an airtight container and store in the refrigerator for up to 3 weeks. Shake well before use.

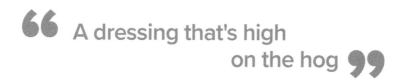

66 A dressing that's high on the hog 99

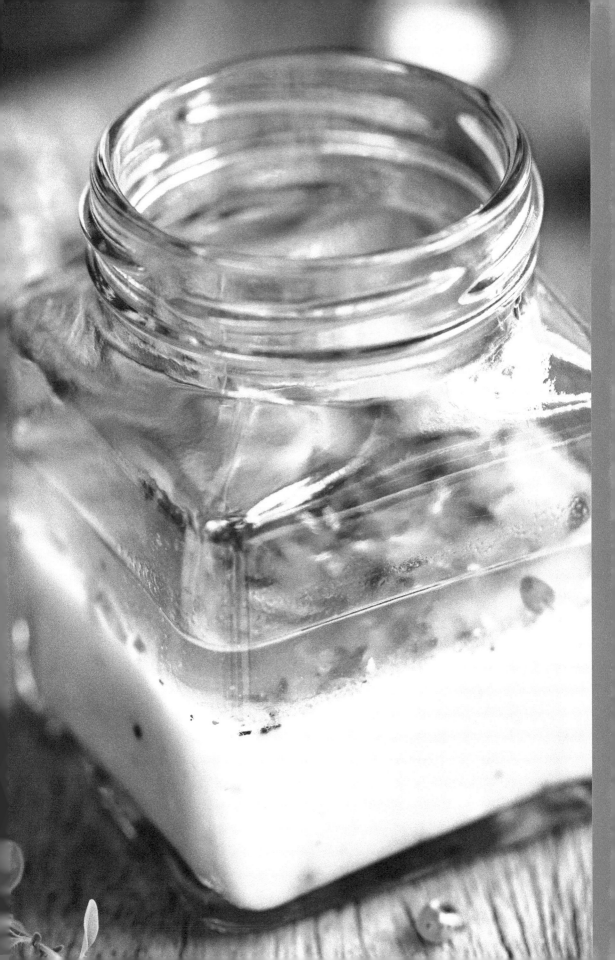

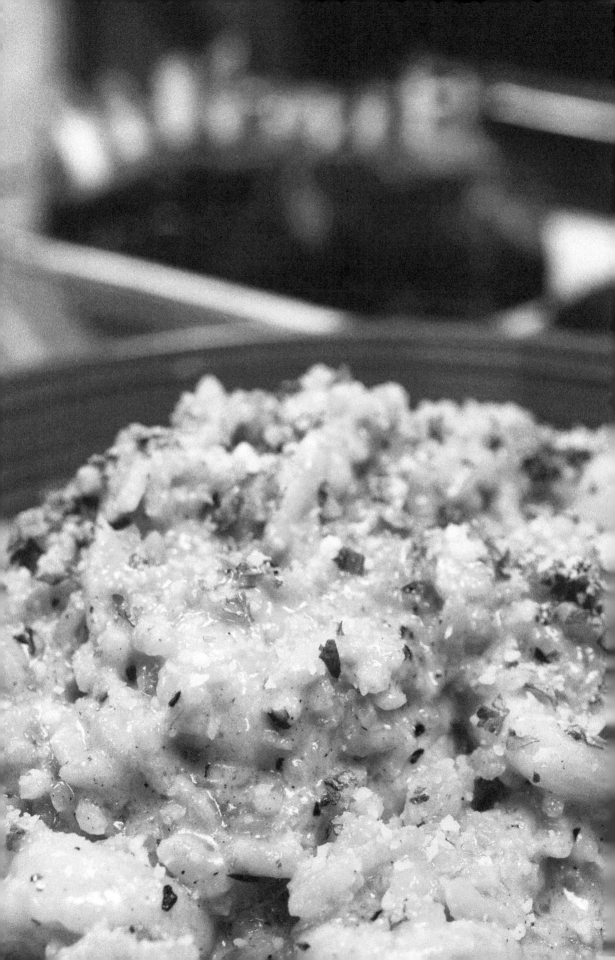

SHRIMP RISOTTO

Serves: 4

INGREDIENTS

2 Tablespoons of unsalted butter

1 Shallot *(chopped)*

1 Teaspoon of dry thyme

1 Teaspoon of cracked
black pepper

1 Cup of Italian rice *(risotto)*

2 ½ Cups of chicken broth

½ Pound of jumbo shrimp
(16/20, peeled, deveined, tail off)

½ Cup of heavy cream

2 Tablespoons of
parmesan cheese

2 Sprigs of fresh dill

DIRECTIONS

Place a large skillet onto the stove on medium high. Add the butter, shallots, thyme and pepper. Sauté for about 4 minutes. Add the rice to the skillet and mix well. Continue cooking for about 2 minutes while stirring constantly. Add the chicken broth one cup at a time. Reduce the heat to medium and continue to stir. Once the broth is totally dissolved, add the remaining broth and continue cooking.

This process should take about 20 minutes. Add the shrimp and cream. Cook for about 5 minutes more. Stir in the cheese. Remove the skillet from the stove and serve. Garnish with fresh dill. Enjoy!

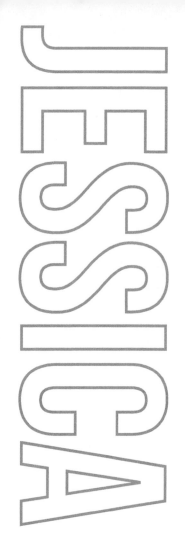

JESSICA

Growing up, I never knew how to cook. I set my frozen waffles on fire once and from there, my parents didn't think it was a good idea for me to use the kitchen anymore. But then I started baking at the Center. I found that it made me feel good.

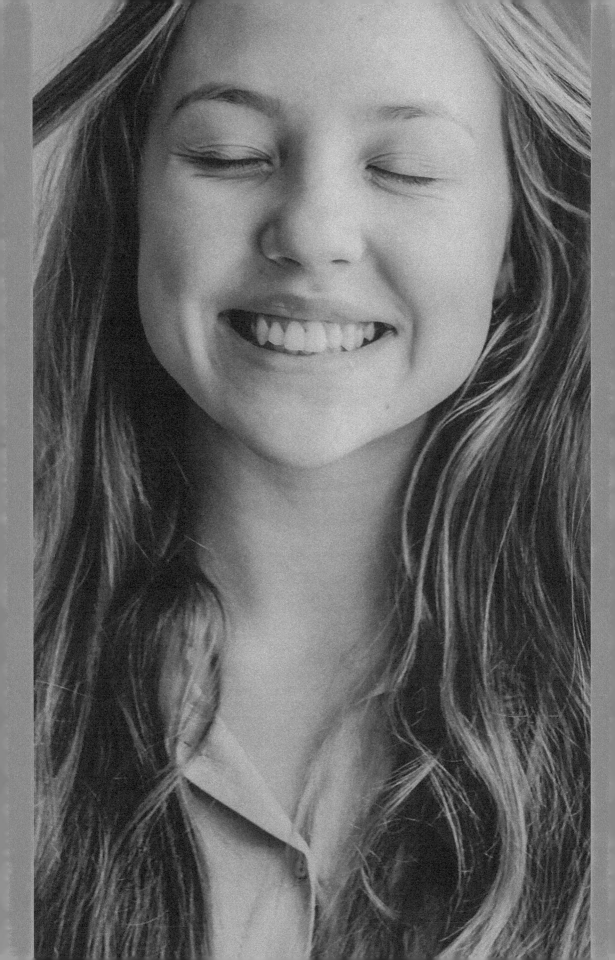

JESSICA

During my childhood, I never learned how to cook. My parents no longer considered it a good idea for me to use the kitchen after I set fire to my frozen waffles one time! This all changed when I started baking at the Center. This activity made me feel good," says Jessica, a 20-year-old student who dreams of working someday in a cupcake bakery.

Among Jessica's diagnoses is "emotional disturbance," which refers to a long-term pattern of behavior that adversely impacts academic performance in children. Jessica has sometimes experienced an out of balance world, but she has always been able to prepare something to make people smile and feel peaceful about herself when she makes people look forward to eating her baked goods. "When I was feeling anxious, Ms. Z brought me to the kitchen, where we began to bake. As Jessica scooped the little balls of dough onto the cookie sheet, her darkness had begun to fade. Pour. Measure. Stir. Jessica was over the attack.

Jessica has suffered from various levels of anxiety for most of her life, but she also suffers from depression, which has always overshadowed her anxiety. In the past year, Blue Cross Blue Shield awarded us a grant for behavioral health support for families affected by the recent pandemic. There is always going to be that need. Our organization raises funds to ensure that students receive the best possible level of support and to identify solutions to improve the problems that negatively impact students. This is a social justice fight we are on board with. Funding allows us to provide parents with the most beneficial mental health solutions possible to help their families thrive. At the Center, we utilize meditation, yoga, healing circles, music, and art therapy, as well as social work groups for stress management. While some of these therapies work well for the students, others, such as Jessica, require a more creative approach and the kitchen is an ideal place to flex that muscle.

66 Among Jessica's diagnoses is *"emotional disturbance,"* which refers to a long-term pattern of behavior that adversely impacts academic performance in children. Jessica has sometimes experienced an out of balance world, but she has always been able to prepare something to make people smile and feel peaceful about herself when she makes people look forward to eating her baked goods. **99**

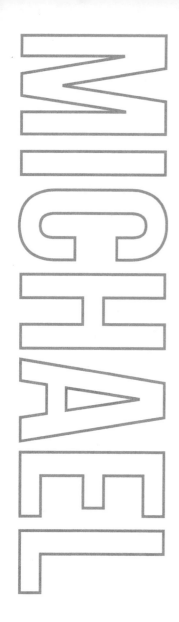

MICHAEL

The bad news about PTSD
is that it does not go away
over time and only gets
worse. The good news is
it responds very well to
treatment.

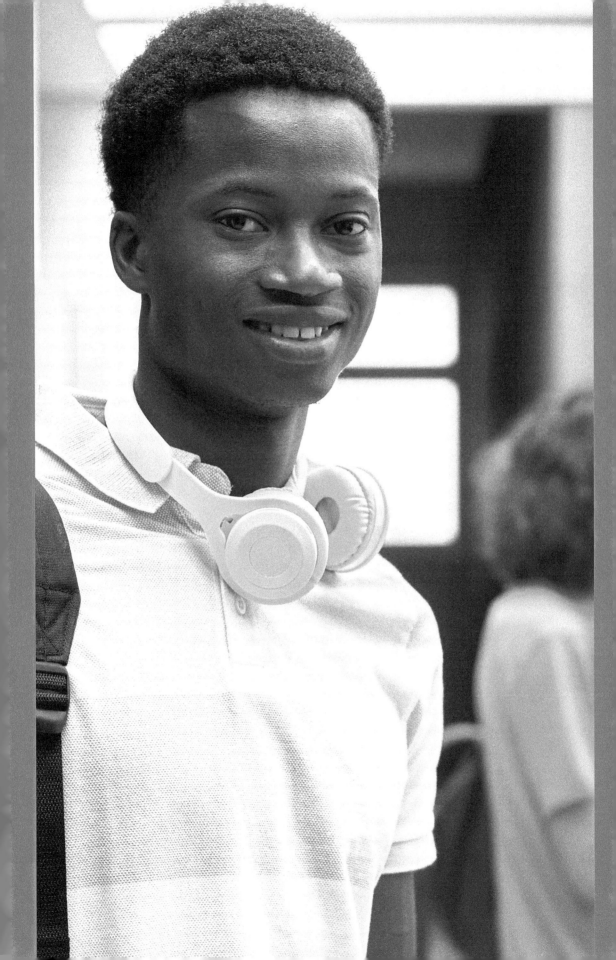

MICHAEL

Michael watched in horror as his best friend was shot to death in front of his school when he was 15 years old. As a 17-year-old high school junior who enjoys anime and video games, Michael came to iCan Dream Center for assistance with social and emotional issues.

Michael's teacher wished that Michael had arrived at the Center sooner after the tragic death of his friend. This young man did not receive the assistance he needed following the shooting to process what he had been through and to grieve for his tragic loss. The team quickly discovered that Michael suffered from post-traumatic stress disorder. Those with the disorder notice every little noise, are easily startled, and are constantly on edge. They are always alert to danger and hypervigilant, so it is extremely difficult to relax. A common complaint is sleep disturbances, along with irritability, anger outbursts, and difficulty concentrating.

When a student is edgy, moody, reactionary, and plum exhausted, the conditions for getting in trouble with authority figures at school present themselves perfectly. PTSD is a chronic illness that does not go away with time. It only gets worse over time. Fortunately, it responds very well to treatment. "Michael, like many of the children we see, just did not have the support from family to cope with his loss, which exasperated his PTSD," says his social worker. Despite this, the kitchen table is an equal playing field.

Everyone has a story. But some of our students don't have that outlet to tell it or adults to tell it for them. Most parents understand the importance of telling their children their story repeatedly so that they can learn who they are and where they belong. At the iCan Dream table, we do this for each other. At the beginning of the pandemic, when images of overcrowded hospitals and death tolls flooded the news, many parents sought refuge in their kitchens by preparing meals for their families. "We sat around the dinner table while the children were listening to their father and I discussing the news," said a principal from one of our partner school districts. "In spite of our lack of understanding, we tried our best to reassure our kids that they were loved and that we would do whatever we could to keep them safe." Kitchen tables can be an intimate sacred healing space. The power of a family meal around the kitchen table to heal the woes of the world simply cannot be overlooked. By bringing them into the kitchen, we provide them with a sense of security, belonging, and safety. What might appear as youngsters standing around making soup is satisfying a human need as essential as food, the need for love.

When Michael left the iCan Dream Center at age 22, he said, "These people became like my family. This was something I had never experienced before. The experience felt good."

66 These people became like my family. This was something I had never experienced before. The experience felt good. **99**

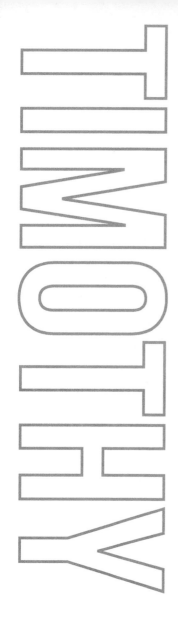

TIMOTHY

The intersectionality of disability, trauma, and food insecurity is a significant barrier for our students and causes us to shift our priorities at times to advocacy and social justice reforms.

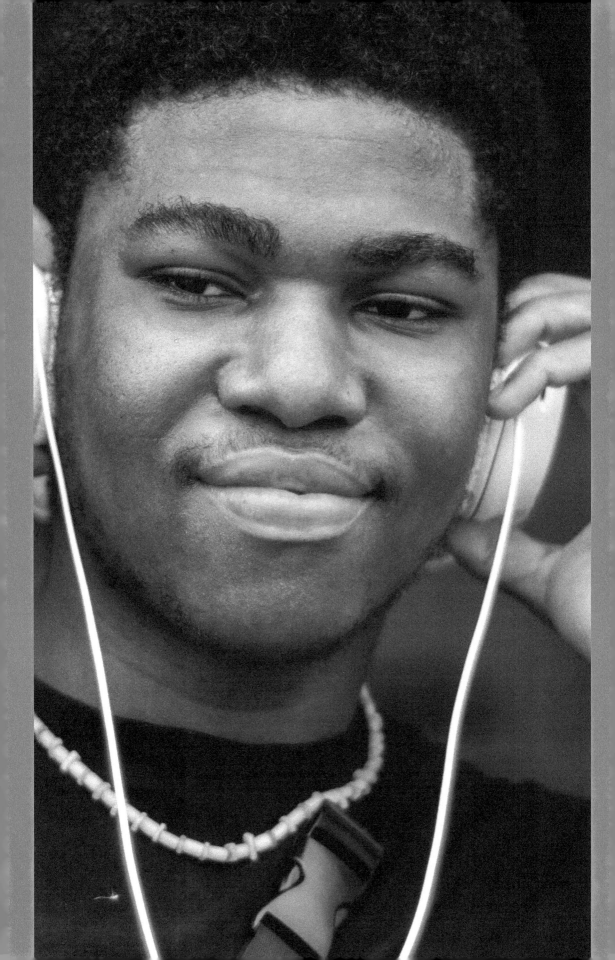

TIMOTHY

Timothy, a 20-year-old young man in our program, is an extremely kind individual. The moment one of our team members learned that Timothy had difficulty eating in the home, he began to imagine the impact this reality would have not just on Timothy's day-to-day struggle, but also on the long-term damage food insecurity would have on Timothy.

Timothy, despite the efforts of our social workers to shield him from pain, still experiences hunger, fatigue, weakness, worry, sadness, and anger due to his awareness of a shortage of food and a resulting lack of food of good quality and quantity.

Individuals experiencing food insecurity have higher rates of mental health problems, including depression, anxiety, and post-traumatic stress disorder. In recent years, growing evidence has linked food insecurity with adverse childhood experiences. Due to the distressing and debilitating nature of food insecurity, as well as the physical and mental health consequences of it, we argue that food insecurity has traumatic implications for young people like Timothy.

A food desert is present in Robbins, Illinois, one of Chicagoland's most depressed communities, where Timothy lives. Timothy's teachers and social workers fill in the gaps by taking him to local food pantries, sending him home with food from the Center, and empowering him by teaching him how to prepare food at home.

There is a complex issue here; our students have intellectual and neurodiverse learning requirements. As a result of the intersectionality of disability, trauma, and food insecurity, we are often forced to shift our priorities to advocacy and social justice reform attempts. The importance of culinary training for Timothy and others like him cannot be overstated. Timothy must know what to do when he gets home with a fresh box of produce or a whole chicken from the food pantry.

Students learn how to peel a potato, boil water, and safely pour it into the sink in culinary class. Timothy is taught how to sanitize the counter and his hands after handling meat, as well as what to do when there is no soap available. Even a little bit of shampoo and hot water will suffice.

Our social workers and teachers see families struggling to find food on a regular basis. In addition to this challenge, there may be other problems in the home or neighborhood, such as unemployment or mental illness. In many cases, their focus becomes very narrow, often focusing on: "How am I going to feed my children? Is there a way to deal with this situation? What am I going to do?" What we like to think makes us unique is our desire to wrap the family in support. From offering parents the opportunity to access free job training at the Center through our Certified Nursing Assistant program to providing parents with behavioral health support to deal with their own trauma, we are constantly looking for ways we can do our part to help restore the family.

"I feel pretty good about my ability to prepare food for myself, but I have a lot to learn about self-care, and I am afraid of going out alone," Timothy says. Ms. Zipporah assures him that he will never be alone.

66 I feel pretty good about my ability to prepare food for myself, but I have a lot to learn about self-care, and I am afraid of going out alone **99**

Put up your hair,
Wash your hands,
Tie your apron strings, nice and snug.
The food you make is like giving a hug.

Read the directions,
Gather your ingredients, and check them twice,
Your food will turn out especially nice.

Follow the directions,
Mix, stir or whisk,
Put your food in a bowl, pan or dish
Whatever the recipe calls for, it is sure to be delish!

Follow directions once again:
It is time to bake, freeze or chill,
Set the timer, Put your recipe where it belongs,
You have got this, you are strong!

While your recipe is baking, freezing or chilling
Clean up the kitchen and make it sparkle,
Your parents will be proud, your family will marvel.
It's time to eat what you have created, Have everyone be seated.

Enjoy the pride you feel for what you have accomplished,
Enjoy the smiles as everyone enjoys the meal they just finished.

Now you know you can take care of you, your friends and your family too!
With the skills you have learned while making this book,
You will never be hungry, because you know how to cook!

By : Peggy Burnap
1958 - 2021

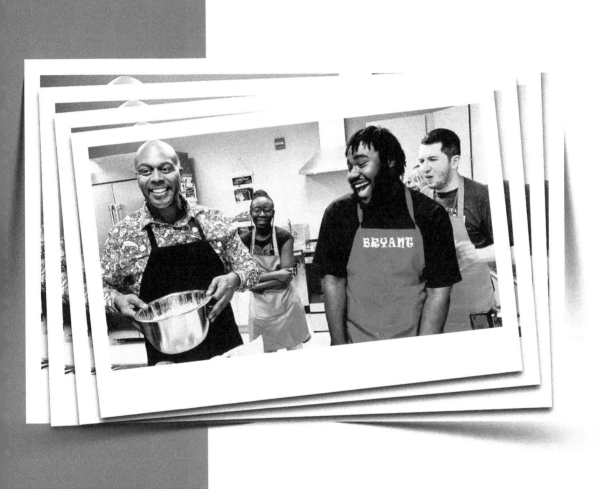

SPICE

and

SPEC TRUM

RECIPES FOR
Resilience

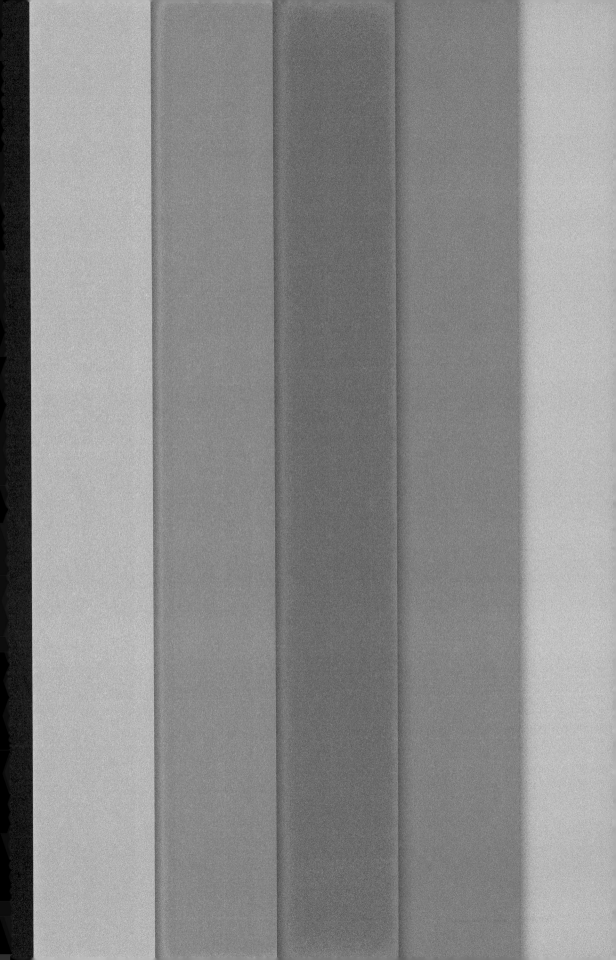

CPSIA information can be obtained
at www.ICGtesting.com
Printed in the USA
JSHW012029181122
33407JS00002B/5